THE ECONOMIC EVOLUTION OF
AMERICAN HEALTH CARE

THE ECONOMIC EVOLUTION OF
AMERICAN HEALTH CARE

FROM MARCUS WELBY
TO MANAGED CARE

David Dranove

PRINCETON UNIVERSITY PRESS   PRINCETON AND OXFORD

Published by Princeton University Press, 41 William Street,
Princeton, New Jersey 08540
In the United Kingdom: Princeton University Press,
3 Market Place, Woodstock, Oxfordshire OX20 1SY
All Rights Reserved

Library of Congress Cataloging-in-Publication Data
Dranove, David.
The economic evolution of American health care : from
Marcus Welby to managed care / David Dranove.
p.   cm.
Includes bibliographical references and index.
ISBN 0-691-06693-8 (alk. paper)
1. Managed care plans (Medical care)—Economic aspects—United
States.   2. Medical care—Economic aspects—United States.
3. Public health—Economic aspects—United States.   I. Title.
RA413.D73 2000
338.4′73621′0973—dc21   00-039975   CIP

This book has been composed in Bauer Bodoni

The paper used in this publication meets the minimum requirements
of ANSI/NISO Z39.48-1992 (R 1997) (*Permanence of Paper*)

www.pup.princeton.edu

Printed in the United States of America

1   3   5   7   9   10   8   6   4   2

Contents

_____ *Acknowledgments* _____

I would like to thank Paul Biondi and Madeleine Shalowitz for conducting extensive background research. I am especially grateful to my wife for letting me bounce ideas off of her, no matter how serious or silly. Lastly, I owe a deep debt of gratitude to Alain Enthoven, who twenty years ago encouraged me to use the lens of economics to bring some clarity to the way we think about health care. I hope this book fits the bill.

THE ECONOMIC EVOLUTION OF
AMERICAN HEALTH CARE

Introduction

FOR THE PAST two decades, I have researched the role of market forces in health care. As a graduate student, I was privileged to study under Alain Enthoven, one of the leading architects of the managed care revolution. Since then, I have been on the faculty of two outstanding business schools. I have always been a big believer in the benefits of competition.

In this book I use an economic lens to examine the historical development of managed care. The starting point for this analysis is the "shopping problem." Economists have long recognized that it is very difficult for patients to shop for medical care. Patients have poor information about what care is needed and where to buy it and also have muted incentives to shop for the best price. The result is that patients are unlikely to be cost-effective medical decision makers. The evolution of the health economy, from the traditional system centered on autonomous physicians, through government planning efforts to today's managed care organizations, represents an ongoing effort to help patients solve the shopping problem.

When I started to write this book, I fully expected it to be a sweeping endorsement of managed care. Indeed, I find a lot of evidence that managed care is working. By one credible estimate, managed care is saving patients over $300 billion annually. At the same time, there is no systematic evidence that managed care has harmed quality. Finally, managed care has clearly won the market test, with the vast majority of privately insured patients enrolled in some type of managed care plan. But managed care has utterly failed to win the trust of American patients and is a favorite target of politicians on both sides of the political spectrum. Piece by piece, politicians may legislate managed care out of existence.

Patients do not trust managed care because they see it as an unnecessary intrusion into the traditional physician-patient relationship. One of my goals in writing this book has been to detail the strengths and weaknesses of the traditional relationship. Another is to refocus the public debate about managed care. The current, simplistic view is that managed care is a cost containment mechanism run amok. The simplistic solution is regulation. I believe that the market forces unleashed by managed care offer opportunities to vastly improve upon the traditional health economy by simultaneously improving quality and containing cost.

In the eighteen months since I began this book, my optimistic view of managed care's potential has wavered. I accept the possibility that managed care will never fulfill its promise. But the problems with managed care come mainly from the outside. I have no doubt that market forces can enable patients to obtain the highest quality care at low prices, while encouraging providers to be efficient and innovative. But I see several hurdles, largely beyond the control of managed care organizations, that must be overcome before we reach this state of health care nirvana:

- Markets have to remain competitive, free of the power struggles emerging between large buyers and providers. This will require vigorous enforcement of antitrust laws.
- There will need to be substantial improvements in health care data. We need better outcomes measures and must be able to link patient-level medical records across providers. This may necessitate government intervention, both to coordinate the collection of data and to establish a confidential patient "identifier."
- Providers must accept that quality varies and must actively engage in quality measurement. Quality measurement is imperfect and unfair to many providers, but providers should rally behind the quality movement because patients stand to benefit.
- Patients must become consumers, willing to shop around for the best managed care plans and the best providers. Patients have much to gain by doing so, perhaps their very lives.

It seems to me that these are all necessary conditions for managed care to be successful. If even one hurdle remains standing, patients will fail to realize the full potential of a truly competitive health economy.

While this seems like a lot to overcome, I remain cautiously optimistic. Despite ongoing merger activity on both the provider and the buyer sides of the market, most urban health care markets remain competitive, and antitrust agencies continue to fight against blatantly anticompetitive combinations. There are massive public and private sector efforts to create sophisticated health care data systems. Providers are gradually getting used to quality evaluation, and patients are increasingly using quality data. We can expect to see more and better data in the future.

My optimism is tempered by the knowledge that improving data and changing attitudes will not happen overnight. In the meantime, patients are growing impatient with organizations that seem to do a better job of managing costs than managing care. Seeking to appeal to angry voters, legislators will enact laws that undo the potential of managed care.

Part One

THE RISE OF MANAGED CARE

CHAPTER 1

Marcus Welby Medicine

MOST BABY BOOMERS remember the popular 1960s television show *Marcus Welby, M.D.* Portrayed by Robert Young, the television doctor was everyone's favorite primary care physician (PCP). He was wise, kind, and one of the most trusted members of his community.[1] He was also at the center of a medical care system not unlike what patients in the real world experienced.

In the era of "Marcus Welby medicine," a patient who fell ill would visit the PCP's private medical office. If the patient could not travel, the PCP might even make a house call. The PCP would spend as much time as necessary to make an initial diagnosis and recommend a treatment. If the patient was not too ill, the PCP would send him or her home with a word of encouragement (and a carefully described prescription, if necessary) and might even phone later to check on the recovery. If the patient was seriously ill, the PCP would make a referral to a specialist or suggest that the patient be admitted to the local nonprofit community hospital. The PCP remained a staunch advocate for the patient throughout treatment.

The PCP and specialists had unquestioned authority within the hospital and retained nearly total control over medical decision making. They merely had to ask, and they would gain access to the hospital's complete arsenal of medical personnel and equipment. Hospital administrators stayed out of medical decision making. They staffed the hospitals, procured supplies, and handled fiscal matters but otherwise deferred to the medical staff in all clinical matters. Nor did health insurers intervene. They sold indemnity insurance, which permitted patients to receive care from any licensed provider, and paid for all services rendered, except possibly for a nominal copayment. With administrators and insurers playing passive roles, physicians clearly stood atop the hierarchy of the health care economy.

In the past two decades, the medical care system embodied by Marcus Welby has disappeared, replaced by one that often seems dispassionate and depersonalized. Nowadays, a patient visits the medical office of a group practice, where the allied medical personnel greatly outnumber the PCPs. After a long wait, the patient spends the majority of time with a nurse or nurse-practitioner. The PCP often does little more than confirm the nurse's diagnosis and dispatch the patient with a hastily written prescription. Nor is the PCP likely to follow up with a phone call after the patient returns home. If the patient is very ill, the PCP might make a referral to a specialist (always in writing to conform to the rules of managed care organizations [MCOs]) but often will consider the financial implications first. After all, many MCOs provide financial rewards to PCPs who limit their referrals. (MCO critics state the converse: MCOs punish PCPs who fail to limit their referrals.)

The demise of the traditional health care system has also affected physician autonomy over medical decision making. Hospital administrators, facing declining reimbursements from Medicare, Medicaid, and MCOs, may force physicians to follow treatment guidelines designed to cut costs. Even worse in the eyes of the medical community, the MCOs themselves are looking over physicians' shoulders. MCOs may refuse to pay for prescription drugs or other services deemed unnecessary, experimental, or too costly. Even if an MCO covers the service, it may force the patient to receive it from an unfamiliar provider. Most infuriating to many patients, most MCOs limit their choice of PCP.

MCOs impose these restrictions largely to save money. In this respect they have been very successful. After three decades of double-digit annual increases in health care expenditures, health care costs are largely under control. Private sector costs were nearly flat for much of the 1990s, and even the recent 6 to 8 percent annual increases in private health insurance premiums are below historical rates of inflation. As documented later in this book, the consensus from the research literature is that these cost savings have been achieved without any systematic reduction in the quality of care. In fact, some MCOs have become catalysts for quality improvement. Americans don't believe it, and MCOs have become among the most unpopular organizations in the United States. Responding to a Harris Company survey in April 1999, American adults ranked MCOs alongside the tobacco industry on service to customers, and only 37 percent felt that MCOs would "do the right thing" if they had a serious problem.[2] Americans may despise MCOs, but they do not display their displeasure in the one place it counts the most—the market. MCOs dominate the health economy, and few patients seem willing to pay the substantially higher price for traditional indemnity insurance.

THE SHOPPING PROBLEM

The transition from Marcus Welby to managed care has been remarkable. In less than thirty years, the American health care system has evolved from one in which patients placed complete trust in their PCPs to one in which they delegate responsibility for life-and-death decisions to individuals and institutions they know little about and trust even less. These two systems for delivering care may seem to have little in common, but I believe they emerged for the same reason. Both represent efforts to solve the fundamental problem of the health economy:

> The fundamental problem of the health economy is that it is difficult for any person or any organization, be they patient, physician, MCO, or the government, to be an efficient and effective purchaser of health care goods and services.

A moment's reflection indicates the enormity of the shopping problem. A patient must determine *what* medical services to buy and *where* to buy them. In addition, the patient must assure the *coordination* of a seemingly endless array of caregivers, including doctors, nurses, hospitals, and outpatient facilities. On their own, most patients lack the knowledge to perform these tasks well. Even a patient who assiduously searches the World Wide Web may, at best, determine what to buy. But that patient is unlikely to find the best place to buy services and will still be left with the challenge of coordinating delivery. It is no wonder that patients have relied on others to do these things for them.

Before the rise of managed care, physicians were almost solely responsible for solving the shopping problem. Patients delegated all authority to physicians and in return obtained what they perceived to be high-quality, care, though at a high cost. In the 1970s, patients tolerated federal and state regulatory efforts to rein in costs, but these regulations failed. Managed care, which began at the start of the century but did not come to dominate the health economy until the 1990s, represents a different solution to the patient's shopping problem, one that emphasizes cost containment and elimination of unnecessary services. But patients do not trust managed care to provide high-quality, and providers protest the heavy hand of MCO intervention. As a result, the shopping problem remains largely unsolved.

Arrow's Argument

In 1963, economist Kenneth Arrow (an eventual Nobel Prize winner) published a landmark paper about the economics of health care.[3] Arrow had just completed pathbreaking research about competitive markets, but in this paper he observes that the way that patients shop for health care services does not resemble shopping behavior in any other markets he had studied. He wonders, for example, why there is no counterpart to the PCP in any other market.

To answer this and other questions, Arrow applies an economic concept called the "survivor principle," which states that any institution or way of doing business that dominates a market must achieve its success by providing greater value to consumers than the alternatives. In applying the survivor principle, Arrow points out that there were alternatives to the traditional health care system that could have emerged but did not. Rather than visiting PCPs to initiate treatment, patients might have directly sought out specialty and hospital care. Physicians could have been employed by hospitals, rather than work directly for patients. For that matter, insurers could have employed physicians. Patients might even have self-diagnosed their illnesses and developed their own treatment plans. In this case, physicians would be little more than technicians providing the requested treatments.

Arrow reasons that if Marcus Welby medicine won the "market test"— that is, if it was the dominant model for organizing health care delivery— then it must have been the superior solution to the shopping problem. Arrow concludes that patients must be better off delegating medical decision-making responsibility to autonomous physicians rather than trying to solve the shopping problem themselves or relying on physician/employees. Arrow then speculates about what it is about health care that makes this so.

SOLVING THE SHOPPING PROBLEM

Arrow observes that when consumers go shopping, whether for groceries, clothing, or dry cleaning, they usually have some idea about what they want to buy. Not so when shopping for medical care. Medicine is complex. Even the most innocent of symptoms, such as hiccups or shortness of breath, can indicate a wide range of diseases, from the mundane to the life-threatening. Very rare is the patient who can confidently self-diagnose the need for a calcium channel blocker, an artificial hip, vascular surgery, or chemotherapy. Of course, there are many other important purchases about which consumers do not know as much as they would like: automobiles, televisions, vacations, computers, college education, retirement investments, and so forth. While consumers often solicit the advice of others about these purchases, they rarely abdicate decision-making authority to the extent that they do when purchasing medical services. To understand why, it is necessary to examine consumer shopping more generally.

In assessing the consumer's shopping problem, economists distinguish between search goods and experience goods. *Search goods* are those for which information about quality or other nonprice dimensions is of virtually no value. Many consumers are indifferent about brands of aspirin, manufacturers of computer diskettes, and retailers of home electronics. For goods and services such as these, quality is not an issue. Instead, consumers select the brand, manufacturer, or retailer largely on the basis of price and convenience. *Experience goods* include those goods and services for which consumers could always stand to have more information. Televisions, automobiles, hairstyling, and lawn maintenance are examples of experience goods. Medical care may be the quintessential experience good; most patients know little, if anything, about their medical care purchases.

Shopping for Experience Goods

Consumers usually do a good job of shopping for experience goods. Diligent consumers have forced electronics firms and automakers to continuously boost quality and reduce costs. Lousy hairstylists and sloppy gardening firms quickly go out of business. How do consumers get the information they need to make well-informed purchases of experience goods? First and foremost, they consider their past experiences with the seller. Consumers also ask friends, coworkers, and relatives about their experiences. At the same time, sellers advertise their products and services, though many consumers are wary of marketing claims. Skeptical consumers often turn to third-party rating services such as *Consumer Reports*. Sometimes consumers cannot obtain information about quality from any of these sources, for example, when such information is hard to describe or when the product is new. In these situations, consumers may rely on the seller's brand name as an indicator of quality. When consumers of cars, high-end stereos, and clothing see the brands BMW, Thiel, and Armani, they know to expect outstanding handling, faithful audio reproduction, and high fashion.

Why Health Care Is Different

When shopping for medical services, patients rarely avail themselves of "traditional" sources of information such as word of mouth or brand name. Instead, they mainly rely upon their physician to shop for them. (A crucial exception, described later, is when patients shop for their PCP.) It follows from the survivor principle that the sources of information that consumers find so useful when shopping for a car or a stereo must be less useful when shopping for medical care. Arrow identified two salient features of health care services that make this so. First, demand for health services is irregular and unpredictable. Second, patient needs are idiosyncratic; that is, no two patients are exactly alike.

Few patients are unfortunate enough to repeatedly purchase the same medical services, especially costly treatments for life-threatening diseases. Nor can many patients predict the need for such services more than a few days or weeks in advance. Lacking both experience and the time to shop around, patients are hard-pressed to develop the expertise necessary to make many important medical purchases. In this way, medical care stands in sharp contrast to other experience goods, such as autos, for which consumers have both substantial experience and ample time to research alternatives.

Unpredictability has a side effect—it fuels the demand for insurance. Patients who lack health insurance are gambling with their wealth. But unlike playing the slots at Las Vegas, this is a gamble that no one enjoys. Health insurance eliminates the gamble, but it makes health care essentially costless to the patient. As we will see later, this has profound implications for the health economy.

Health care needs are not only unpredictable but also highly idiosyncratic. Two patients may have similar symptoms but vastly different conditions. Two patients with the same condition may respond in very different ways to identical treatments. As a result, patients can not rely too heavily on the anecdotal experiences of others when making a self-diagnosis, when evaluating a treatment plan, or even when selecting a provider. Health care has become more specialized over the years, making it more difficult than ever for patients to draw conclusions about their own medical needs on the basis of the experiences of others.

Patients not only have a difficult time determining what medical services to buy but also need help determining where to buy them. When seeking care from specialists and hospitals, patients naturally want the very best. Until the last few years, there was no easy way for patients to quantitatively rank the best hospitals, specialists, or other medical providers. Even today, published rankings of providers are rudimentary, and few patients use them.

Unable to rely on personal experiences, word of mouth, or hard evidence, it is no wonder that patients have relied on their physicians to solve the shopping problem. Who better to turn to than physicians? Physicians spend four years in medical school and another four to six years in residency training, have many additional years of experience, keep up with medical journals, attend conferences and continuing education programs, and regularly network with colleagues. Physicians seem to have the necessary information that patients lack. Assuming that physicians act unselfishly (an assumption I will take up later on), it makes perfect sense for patients to turn over complete decision-making authority to them.

Doctor Web?

Many policy analysts believe that patients need to assume more responsibility for solving the shopping problem.[4] Through the Internet, patients certainly have unprecedented opportunities to do so. There are over twenty thousand medical sites on the World Wide Web, including sites from leading academic institutions like the Mayo Clinic and Johns Hopkins Hospital, as well as profit-seeking organizations such as America's Health Network (formed by Richard Scott, former president of the Columbia/HCA hospital chain). Patients can use these sites to investigate symptoms, find out about prescription drugs, or learn about the latest treatments for what ails them. For example, patients who peruse the Cleveland Clinic's Web site will find easy-to-read reports on literally hundreds of health topics ranging from acromegaly (a hormonal disorder) to yeast infections. Patients can also use the Web to contact others with similar medical conditions, thus forming a worldwide support community.

The Internet empowers patients to take purchasing decisions into their own hands instead of relying utterly on their physicians, but it will not replace the traditional doctor-patient relationship any time soon. Even the best Web sites barely scratch the surface in their descriptions of symptoms and treatments. For example, drkoop.com (started by former surgeon general C. Everett Koop) offers fewer than one thousand words on the treatment and management of diabetes and seven hundred words about migraine headaches. Nor is the information provided by medical Web sites necessarily objective. Pharmaceutical manufacturers pay these sites a lot of money (reportedly in the six figures) for the rights to provide content and hot links to other sites. To make matters worse, different sites often give conflicting information. Some sites recommend adenoidectomy to remove enlarged adenoids, whereas others recommend against it. Some sites recommend H^2-antagonists to treat heartburn; others mention trying antibiotics. The resulting confusion has become a major headache for physicians, many of whom waste time with patients reconciling conflicting information or explaining why information gleaned from the Internet is not relevant to their case. Sometimes physicians have to perform unnecessary tests just to rule out diagnoses that their patients pulled off the Internet.

Despite the wealth of information available on the Internet, it may be harder than ever before for patients to do their own shopping. One reason is that the information can be confusing; another is that there is so much more to know. Medicine is growing more complex every year. The number of journals covered by *Index Medicus* (the leading index of medical journals) increased by 50 percent between 1968 and 1998. For some diseases, the explosion of knowledge is even more rapid, with five- to tenfold increases in the number of published research articles on diseases like angina, diabetes, and breast cancer. One area in which innovation has been particularly noticeable is drug therapy. During the 1960s and 1970s, the Food and Drug Administration approved between fifteen and twenty new drugs per year. It now approves as many as fifty drugs per year, each of which has unique therapeutic benefits, interactions with other drugs, and side effects.[5] Patients must also contend with an increasing pace of innovation in medical devices, surgical procedures, and diagnostic technologies. Thirty years ago, patients could not begin to develop the expertise required to make their own medical decisions. Nowadays, even Marcus Welby might have a hard time keeping up.

Eventually the Internet may help patients ask better questions of their health care providers, but it is doubtful that it will enable patients to bypass their physicians altogether. Patients will continue to rely on their physicians to solve the shopping problem. But this begs two questions. First, how can patients be sure that their physicians will act unselfishly? Second, how can patients be sure they have done a good job of selecting their physician? The answers lie in a more in-depth examination of the shopping problem and the important role of trust.

TRUST AND THE PHYSICIAN-PATIENT RELATIONSHIP

Physician services are experience goods; patients could stand to have a lot of information when shopping for a physician. Is the physician capable? Will the physician act unselfishly? Will the physician do everything possible to effect a cure? These uncertainties are not unique to medicine. There are many situations in which one person, called the *principal*, delegates decision-making authority to another, called the *agent* (in medicine, the patient is the principal and the physician is the agent). It is not unusual for a principal to be uncertain about whether the agent is hardworking, capable, and willing to act in the principal's behalf. Faced with these uncertainties, the principal has two choices: try to use a contract to force the agent to perform as desired or else rely on trust.

Contracts versus Trust

The late James Coleman, a prominent sociologist, described situations involving trust as those "in which the *risk* one takes depends on the performance of another actor."[6] This certainly characterizes the physician-patient relationship, where the health of the patient depends critically on the performance of the physician. Coleman adds that the action of placing trust involves the trustor's voluntarily placing resources at the disposal of another party, without any real commitment from that other party." These real commitments are the essential ingredients of contracts. By implication, contracts are an alternative to trust. Yet the idea of using contracts to bind providers and patients is almost unheard of. Economists have identified a number of limitations of contracting, associated with bounded rationality, hidden action, and hidden information, that make contracts less than ideal for use in medicine.

Bounded rationality refers to the limited ability of individuals to deal with complexity and to precisely define or measure actions and outcomes. As a result of bounded rationality, contracts rarely cover all possible contingencies. *Hidden actions* are those taken by agents that the principal cannot observe. The principal cannot rely on a contract to encourage or prevent hidden actions, and he or she may refuse to contract with the agent if the hidden action can be especially damaging. The principal or agent possesses *hidden information* when the other party does not possess it. When one party knows that the other has "something up its sleeve," it may be reluctant to enter into a contract.

The medical care process and the doctor-patient relationship are replete with bounded rationality, hidden actions, and hidden information. A contract between physician and patient would have to define success and failure. It would therefore need to define sickness and health. It would also need to spell out the various problems that might arise during treatment and sort out those problems that would be the fault of the provider from those that arose for reasons beyond the provider's control. To further confound the contracting problem, patients could take hidden actions (e.g., regular exercise after treatment) that affect outcomes. Patients may also have hidden information (e.g., about other symptoms, or the support of family members) that could affect outcomes. Physicians may also take hidden actions (e.g., take extra time reviewing test results) and may have hidden information (e.g., about the availability of various therapies). For all of these reasons, patients and providers may be unable or unwilling to agree to a contract.

FORMS OF TRUST

Without contracts, patients must rely on trust. Sociologist David Mechanic observes that the trust that patients place in their physicians manifests itself in several forms (1) trust that providers will act unselfishly, putting patients' interests above their own, (2) trust that providers have the technical competence necessary for proper diagnosis and treatment, and (3) trust that providers can control and coordinate the resources necessary to deliver quality care.[7]

Trust in Unselfishness

Mechanic writes, "The public legitimacy of the medical profession rests substantially on the perception of physicians as dedicated patient advocates," and that before the advent of managed care "medicine was viewed as a selfless endeavor."[8] Patients have always expected physicians, especially PCPs, to be deeply concerned about their welfare. They have had no such expectations about most other agents, including plumbers, insurance agents, or even professors. Patients have had good reason to expect physicians to act unselfishly. Prior to the development of antibiotics in the 1940s, physicians often had little else to offer their patients besides compassion.[9] As a result, medicine was a "calling" for those who wanted to comfort the sick and dying. For many physicians, medicine remains a calling. While the financial rewards can be great, money is not the only factor that lures people into the profession. Most of the talented young college students who have chosen to become physicians could have fared equally well financially had they become lawyers or consultants.[10]

Medical school and residency training reinforce the high ideals of dedication and selflessness. Instructors emphasize the importance of placing the medical interests of patients above the fiduciary interests of hospitals and insurance companies. Medical school graduates take the Hippocratic oath, in which they swear, "In every house where I come I will enter only for the good of my patients." As managed care has forced physicians to confront economic trade-offs, medical schools have reaffirmed the Hippocratic ideals. Today, most U.S. medical schools offer a course in medical ethics (which many schools require for graduation), and over a dozen schools have medical ethics or bioethics research centers. Professional associations provide the same message. The American Medical Association (AMA) has developed seven Principles of Medical Ethics, which it describes as a "potent, vigorous contract of caring between physicians and patients." The principles stress dedication, compassion, and responsibility.

Of course, no amount of training can force a physician to behave unselfishly, and such training might even be unnecessary. Some physicians are unselfish by nature. Those who are selfish by nature surely realize that they stand to gain financially by at least appearing to be unselfish. After all, compassion boosts demand. In light of evidence presented throughout this book about how providers respond to financial incentives, it is easy to be cynical and conclude that a physician's good bedside manner is, like Dr. Welby, just an act. But most patients believe that the compassion is genuine. As Mechanic puts it, "Although there was always some threat that economic incentives might induce the physician to prescribe unnecessarily, . . . there was little ambiguity about the expectation that the physician's loyalty was to the patient."[11]

Trust in Competence

I once asked my students to evaluate the abilities of their own PCPs. Were they average, above average, exceptional, or perhaps just mediocre? One of the students, a doctor taking time out from his medical practice to pursue a management degree, was very troubled by the question. He felt that because all physicians must pass certification exams and complete rigorous residency training, they were all, in a sense, "above average." (This was eerily reminiscent of humorist Garrison Keillor's claim about the mythical town of Lake Wobegone, where "all of the children are above average"). I think my student meant that all physicians are capable of providing quality medical care. Most patients would agree and would readily accept the medical advice of almost any physician. But most patients also believe that there is a range of abilities, and, all else being equal, they would naturally gravitate toward the best physicians. Patients with serious illnesses may be particularly likely to seek out the best.

Patients search for the best physicians in somewhat the same way that they search for the best providers of other experience goods: by asking others for advice. They may ask friends and relatives for the name of a good PCP, and they usually turn to their PCP for a referral to a specialist. In addition to these trusted sources of subjective information, patients may ask physicians where they went to medical school. Presumably, patients are more willing to trust a graduate of Johns Hopkins or Northwestern University than a graduate of a less renowned institution. Patients prefer specialists to generalists, and, in the words of comedian Jackie Mason, they seek out the "biggest" specialists. Patients prefer teaching hospitals and physicians affiliated with them. In these ways, educational and hospital affiliations serve the same role in medicine that brand names serve in other markets. In effect, Johns Hopkins becomes the brand.

There is an important difference, however, between the way patients shop for medical care and the way they shop for other experience goods. For all intents and purposes, there is no *Consumer Reports* for medical care. It is not as if quality evaluation is unnecessary. To paraphrase one of the nation's leading health services researchers, Robert Brook, quality variation across providers is "immense."[12] (I will have much more to say about this claim in Chapter 7.) Patients would presumably benefit a good deal if they could identify the best providers, yet they tend to ignore the few independent, objective sources of information about provider quality.

If patients rely on subjective appraisals rather than objective data, how do they know whether they are getting good medical care? I am surprised at how few patients ask this question. Marcus Welby's patients undoubtedly felt that he provided quality care. But what was the basis for their conclusion? Did Dr. Welby's patients take his kindness as evidence of his clinical capabilities? Marcus Welby may have left his patients feeling warm and fuzzy about their medical care, and "warm fuzzies" can certainly contribute toward healing, but there is no substitute for accurate diagnoses, carefully developed treatment plans, and expert implementation of those plans. It is possible that Dr. Welby's patients confused trust in compassion with trust in competence.

Compassion and competence do not necessarily go hand in hand. Consider how these evolved during the 1970s. At that time, prominent observers of the health care system were bemoaning the deterioration of compassion.[13] Senator Edward Kennedy complained about the rise of specialists, Sidney Wolfe (of Ralph Nader's Public Citizen group) criticized the way physicians wrote prescriptions and used machines rather than speaking with their patients, and *Newsweek* argued that medical education was steering young physicians away from "the role of comforter of the sick towards the job of technologist." Kennedy, Wolfe, and *Newsweek* were concerned that physicians no longer seemed to care about their patients. Sociologists Darryl Enos and Paul Sultan concurred, offering the widely held view that somehow the health care system had strayed from its mission of comforting the psyches of the sick.[14] They quote from a 1927 issue of the *Journal of the American Medical Association*: "One of the essential qualities of the clinician is interest in humanity, for the secret of the care of the patient is in caring for the patient." Specialization and the increased reliance on technology certainly seemed to threaten that caring relationship.

But medicine had come a long way between 1927 and 1977. Providers were increasingly able to cure disease, not just care for the symptoms. Rather than tend to the mental state of their patients, physicians could directly attack the root physical causes of their ailments (although it is increasingly recognized that the former can be helpful to the latter). There were dramatic advances in diagnostic imaging, blood testing, and anesthetics. Surgeons were learning how to resection arteries and transplant organs. These advances necessitated intervention by specialists, administration of drugs, and use of costly new machines. As a result, medicine became less personal; physicians became better technicians but had less time for communication; they were more inclined to heal the body than the mind. It seems that even as patients reaffirmed their trust in the competence of providers, they may have started having doubts about their compassion.

Trust in the Ability of Providers to Control and Coordinate Resources

Compassion and competence are not enough to assure the delivery of quality medical care. To treat many illnesses, physicians must harness a wide range of medical resources, from outpatient diagnostic tests to the full arsenal of services offered by tertiary care hospitals, including nursing, physical and occupational therapy, radiology, pathology, intensive care, drugs, and supplies. As economist Victor Fuchs put it, the physician is "the captain of the team."[15] Fuchs adds that the physician "is the gatekeeper to the production of medical care. The actual delivery of care is frequently in the hands of other health professionals—pharmacists, nurses, technicians, and the like—but they take their instructions from the physician and report back to him."[16]

Hospital care is the quintessential situation in which the physician is the team captain. Echoing Fuchs's description of the physician's leadership role, economist Mark Pauly describes the hospital as the "doctor's workshop."[17] Hospital care involves a vast array of highly trained medical professionals, including physicians, nurses, technicians, and therapists. It also involves a wide range of services and technologies, including intensive care, inhalation therapy, magnetic resonance imaging (MRI), and catheters. The attending physicians who take charge of patient care within hospitals make sure that their patients have timely access to the correct people and services. Inappropriate decisions and poor allocation of resources could have dire consequences for the patient.

Patients trust their physicians to control and coordinate the medical resources necessary for high-quality care. Mechanic states, "We take it for granted that the clinician has access to the means to maintain our health."[18] According to economist and physician Jeffrey Harris, "The patient buys a promise from the doctor to be fixed up. The hospital in turn . . . supplies the necessary inputs to the doctor. . . . There is a strong ethical presumption that the doctor be *left alone* to do whatever is necessary for the patient's well-being."[19] According to Harris, this is most likely to occur when physicians are *independent* from the hospitals in which they work.

Physician autonomy has been a defining feature of our health economy for nearly the entire century. Prior to the 1980s, virtually all physicians had a solo practice or belonged to a small group. Although most physicians today belong to groups, most groups remain small; groups with more than fifty physicians are very uncommon. Only a few physicians, such as medical residents, hospital-based RAP physicians (radiologists, anesthesiologists, and pathologists), and physicians in staff-model health maintenance organizations (HMOs), are employees of hospitals or other organizations. Most physicians still work directly for their patients.

Harris argues that by maintaining autonomy, physicians can control and coordinate resources so as to assure the highest possible quality of care. Harris observes that complex problems frequently arise during a hospitalization, leading to critical demands for resources. At these times, inappropriate decisions about what care to provide and when to provide it could be catastrophic. Under these conditions, it makes sense to assign final decision-making authority to physicians rather than an administrator. Physicians have both superior medical knowledge and greater loyalty to their patients. They place more weight on quality than on cost and are less likely to make choices that would jeopardize their patients' health.

NONPROFITS IN THE HEALTH ECONOMY

The patient's shopping problem does not end with the delegation of decision-making authority to trusted, autonomous physicians. Nor does physician autonomy guarantee that physicians will have total control over the medical care process. Managers of hospitals and other health care organizations make important decisions that ultimately contribute to the quality of care. They hire staff and purchase equipment. They arrange for training and assemble treatment teams. Can patients trust health care managers as much as they trust their physicians? Why should they? After all, there is no Hippocratic oath for managers. Perhaps more significantly, many of the organizations they run are owned by profit-seeking investors, and, as Arrow notes, "The very word profit is a signal that denies the trust relations."[20]

If Arrow is correct, an easy way for health care organizations to win the trust of their patients is to set aside the profit motive. Many have done so; nonprofit organizations play a central role in the health economy. Hospitals, which account for about 40 percent of the health economy, are predominantly nonprofit. Nursing homes and other long-term care facilities, which account for about 10 percent of the health economy, are a mix of nonprofits and for-profits, and nonprofits have dominant market shares among non-Medicaid nursing home patients. The health insurance and managed care market is also a mix of nonprofits and for-profits. Many prominent for-profit insurance companies, including Aetna and CIGNA sell health insurance. But some of the largest health insurers, including most of the Blue Cross and Blue Shield plans and the giant Kaiser managed care plans, are nonprofits. Only a few sectors of the health economy, including the prescription drug and medical supply sectors, are dominated by for-profits.

WHY ARE THERE NONPROFITS?

To understand why nonprofits dominate some sectors of the health economy but not others, it is helpful to think broadly about the types of goods and services that nonprofits provide. Some that come to mind are theater productions, food and housing for the homeless, and medical care for the uninsured. These goods and services provide a "community benefit," that is, they benefit the community as a whole. Almost everyone wants these goods and services to be available even if they do not personally plan to use them. People seem to feel better about themselves and their community when the performing arts are prominent, the homeless are fed and sheltered, and the uninsured receive necessary medical care.

Many for-profits offer goods and services that provide a community benefit. There are for-profit theaters and for-profit day care centers, and for-profit hospitals provide some uncompensated care. But for-profits may not do enough. Unless the government directly provides the needed goods and services, communities must rely on nonprofits to fill the void. In the health economy, nonprofits offer a number of services that provide community benefit. Nonprofit hospitals treat the uninsured and offer unprofitable services such as trauma care. Nonprofit Blue Cross and Blue Shield insurance plans offer reduced premiums on health insurance for high-risk enrollees. Without nonprofits, these goods and services might be unavailable. On the other hand, there is no need for nonprofits in the pharmaceutical sector, where private demand is sufficient to assure a steady flow of new drugs to treat a wide range of diseases.

How can nonprofits afford to offer unprofitable services? The conventional wisdom is that nonprofits rely on charitable contributions. But with a few exceptions (such as children's hospitals), most nonprofit health care organizations get very little money from charity, often less than 1 percent of total revenues. To help them survive, the government provides tax breaks, including exemption from local property taxes. For-profits complain, sometimes bitterly, that these tax breaks give nonprofits an unfair competitive advantage. Executives at the for-profit Columbia/HCA hospital chain have even refused to use the label "nonprofit," instead describing nonprofit hospitals as "non-taxpaying" organizations. But the tax breaks do not fully explain how nonprofits survive. One study found that 80 percent of hospitals spend more on community benefits than they receive in tax breaks.[21] There must be something besides tax breaks that enables nonprofits to successfully compete head-to-head against for-profits.

We can understand the success of nonprofits by once again invoking the survivor principle. If nonprofits dominate some sectors of the health economy, it follows from the survivor principle that they must provide greater value to consumers. This must be especially true for hospitals, which are predominantly nonprofit, but less relevant to the medical R&D sector, where for-profits dominate. But what is it about nonprofit hospitals that consumers value? To understand how nonprofits create value, we must again turn to economic theory.

THE THEORY OF NONPROFITS

In most markets, for-profits dominate, and self-interest is an accepted norm. The Nobel Prize–winning economist Milton Friedman once stated that "the social responsibility of business is to increase its profits,"[22] a sentiment echoed by Michael Douglas's character Gordon Gecko in the quintessential 1980s movie *Wall Street*. Gecko's infamous motto was "Greed is good." There is nothing necessarily incompatible between pursuing profits and serving society's interests. Most profit-seeking businesses make money by efficiently producing goods and services that meet consumer needs. Of course, nonprofits also wish to efficiently meet consumer needs. The survivor principle tells us that, in most markets, for-profits do it better. The for-profit pharmaceutical industry has done it so well that even in socialist-leaning northern Europe, pharmaceutical manufacturers are among the leading investor-owned companies.

There are several possible reasons that for-profits dominate most sectors of the economy. Perhaps for-profits attract more talented workers and managers and do a better job of motivating them to work hard. For-profits can issue stocks and options, and they base pay on easily measured metrics such as stock market performance. These high-powered financial incentives may be attractive to top workers and managers, and may motivate them not to shirk. On the other hand, health care can be a calling to workers and managers, not just physicians. As a result, nonprofits may be able to attract their share of talented and self-motivated workers and managers.

Perhaps for-profits use their superior access to capital markets to grow, innovate, and improve efficiency. Nonprofits must rely on debt markets and often must work with government agencies that issue their bonds. This puts a drag on their access to capital. Quick access to equity capital (i.e., stock) enables for-profits to more rapidly expand into new markets, launch new creative ventures, or reorganize in the face of operational inefficiencies. It is doubtful, for example, that Amazon.com could have rapidly expanded its product line and distribution network without its quick access to equity capital.

The ability of nonprofits to attract good managers partially explains why nonprofits are able to keep up with for-profits. But given the for-profit advantage in attracting capital, one wonders how nonprofits can outperform for-profits. Nonprofit supporters say the key is quality.

Nonprofits and Quality

Certainly, quality is more important in the health economy than in most other sectors of the economy. But other markets where consumers demand high quality, such as the automobile market, are dominated by for-profits. The difference is not so much whether consumers want high quality but whether they can figure out if they are getting it. When consumers are well-informed about quality, the profit motive works to their advantage. They can patronize those firms that best meet their needs. The problem is that profit-driven sellers may provide the wrong products, at substandard quality, *in those markets where it is difficult for consumers to evaluate their own needs and quality is hard to measure.* This is why patients trust their PCPs to help them make the right purchasing decisions. But patients cannot be certain that their PCPs will make the best choices, and patients make some choices on their own, such as when they select a nursing home. It seems that patients can use additional assurance when assessing their needs and selecting a provider. They might prefer a provider whom they believe is unlikely to take advantage of them. Nonprofit providers fit the bill.[23]

The Nonprofit "Assurance"

With few exceptions, nonprofit firms may not distribute their earnings to managers or owners. A "charitable" nonprofit that violates this restriction faces fines and the loss of its tax-exempt status.[24] Unable to personally prosper from their firms' profits, managers of charitable nonprofits presumably have less incentive to cut costs by reducing quality.

To illustrate how this difference in incentives plays out in practice, consider the use of catheters. U.S. health care providers use 200 million catheters annually. Providers can employ a variety of techniques to assure the safe use of catheters, including the purchase of "safety catheters," which, among other things, are impossible to reuse. But these can cost five times more than standard catheters. We might expect profit-driven managers to back off on this expense, reasoning that patients would never find out what kinds of catheters are used.[25] Nonprofit managers, who are less likely to hew to the bottom line, might be more likely to consider incurring these expenses.

Hospitals and other health care organizations have many other opportunities to shirk on quality in ways that patients cannot easily detect. Here are just a few examples:

- *Staffing levels.* Does the hospital have enough nurses, technicians, and other personnel on staff to assure timely, continuous care, or are the staff spread so thinly that quality is compromised? Unless patients have enough experience to know what the "right" level of staffing is, they are unlikely to detect a staffing shortage unless it becomes serious.
- *Staff training.* Does the hospital rely excessively on nurse aides to perform tasks that should be done by registered nurses? Is the medical staff certified in the appropriate specialties? Patients are unlikely to check up on credentialing and even less likely to know what constitutes appropriate credentialing.
- *Equipment.* Does the hospital use state-of-the-art equipment that is well maintained, or does it use outdated, faulty equipment that limits diagnostic accuracy and therapeutic quality? Patients would be at a loss to determine if the medical equipment is appropriate and functioning properly.
- *Utilization.* The hospital may cut back on services to hold down costs and boost profits. Patients may not know the correct level of services and therefore may not figure out if they are being short-changed.

Patients who cannot evaluate these *hard-to-measure attributes* might reasonably believe that nonprofits will place quality above profits. This gives nonprofits the edge they need to survive in competitive markets.

Are Nonprofits Really Nonprofit?

The theory of nonprofits states that they will not exploit their uninformed consumers by shirking on quality. But in several studies published in the 1970s, economists suggest that nonprofits do not always serve the interests of consumers. For example, Joseph Newhouse and others speculate that nonprofit managers overinvest in staffing and costly medical technology to maximize their prestige.[26] Mark Pauly and Mark Redisch posit that nonprofit hospital managers give de facto control to physicians, who run the hospitals to maximize their own incomes.[27] (Note how this theory ascribes the profit motive to physicians.) Through these and other arguments, many have wondered if nonprofits are any different than for-profits. As one letter writer to the trade magazine *Hospitals* put it: "Don't tell me a nonprofit hospital doesn't make a profit. The only answer is that none of the profit goes to any member of the board, etc. And if a nonprofit hospital is not making a profit, something is wrong with the management."[28]

If nonprofits are making a profit, what do their managers do with it? Invest in expensive equipment so as to maximize prestige? Turn the profits over to physicians? Purchase mahogany desks and attend seminars in the south of France? There is probably a little bit of each going on, but I doubt if there is a lot. If there was, one would wonder why a church or community organization would establish a nonprofit hospital. I think it is reasonable to conclude that managers of nonprofits want to serve their communities. Even so, they must first assure the financial viability of their organizations. Sometimes this means that managers must emphasize the bottom line.

Many nonprofit providers operate in fiercely competitive markets, and, as a result, their managers face difficult choices. They can pursue charitable goals but jeopardize the financial health of the organization, or they can mimic the actions of for-profits but fall short on fulfilling the nonprofit mission. Nonprofit managers are likely to strike a balance between the two. As long as the organization's finances are healthy, managers can pursue unprofitable activities that fulfill the mission, while maintaining prices below what the market will bear. But if the organization's finances are not healthy, the mission may have to take a backseat to financial considerations. At the same time, managers may have to increase prices closer to the profit-maximizing level. This is known as "cost-shifting."

Cost-Shifting

Until the early 1980s, the managers of nonprofit health care organizations were under little financial pressure. Market conditions enabled even badly managed hospitals to survive. Private insurers either paid whatever price the hospital charged or paid the hospital for its costs plus a predetermined profit margin. Government insurers—Medicare and Medicaid—also paid on a cost-plus basis.[29] As a result, hospitals that boosted quality could count on getting reimbursed for most or all of the expense. Those that provided unprofitable services or cared for the uninsured covered the expenses by charging higher prices to everyone else.

The idea that hospitals could raise prices to their privately insured patients to generate the revenues necessary to pursue their mission became known as "cost-shifting." Insurers first worried about cost-shifting in the early 1970s, when some state Medicaid programs reduced their payments to hospitals. Hospitals responded by raising prices to privately insured patients.[30] Concern about cost-shifting intensified in the early 1980s, as more states cut their Medicaid payments. In 1984, the Health Insurance Association of America (HIAA), which represents mainly small indemnity insurers, claimed that shortfalls in public sector funding were causing hospitals to shift nearly $9 billion annually onto private payers. The HIAA called for increases in Medicare and Medicaid payments.

Recent research suggests that managed care has put an end to cost-shifting.[31] A hospital that raises its prices to make up for cutbacks in government payments risks exclusion from managed care networks. For example, William White and I find that the hospitals hardest hit by Medicaid cutbacks actually lowered prices to privately insured patients, apparently in an effort to increase managed care enrollments. Unable to cost-shift, hospitals must find other ways to cope. We find that hospitals reduced service levels and, in the extreme, closed. In a related study, Jon Gruber finds that hospitals in competitive markets have cut back on charity care.[32]

WHAT DO THE FACTS SHOW ABOUT NONPROFITS?

There has been considerable research about the differences in quality between nonprofit and for-profit providers. The findings are mixed. An Institute of Medicine report from 1986 finds no consistent evidence of lower quality at for-profit hospitals, but it does find that "most studies on quality of nursing home care tend to favor the not-for-profit mode."[33] Nonprofits tended to have better staffing and better food and were more likely to comply with regulations. Almost all of the worst nursing homes were for-profits.

In his studies of nursing homes and facilities for the mentally handicapped, Burton Weisbrod focuses on hard-to-measure attributes such as the use of sedatives and periodic review of patient needs.[34] He finds that church-owned nonprofits are particularly more likely to provide higher levels of these attributes. Weisbrod also finds that private-paying patients endure long waiting lists for admission to nonprofits. Private-paying patients have immediate access to for-profits, which tend to admit mostly patients covered by Medicaid. This supports the view that consumers believe that nonprofits offer superior quality, even if they cannot measure it.

A study team led by Frank Sloan examines patient outcomes and finds that Medicare patients undergoing major surgery at nonprofit hospitals and for-profit hospitals had similar two-year survival probabilities: 69 percent at for-profits and 67 percent at nonprofits.[35] Although this difference of 2 percentage points may be large enough to cause concern among patients and policy makers, the margin for error in Sloan's estimates is roughly 5 percentage points, so it is not statistically meaningful.

One recent study suggests that for-profit MCOs deliver a lower quality of care than nonprofits.[36] The study compares a number of quality indicators, including immunization rates, prenatal care rates, and administration of beta-blockers following myocardial infarction. For-profits consistently scored lower on these indicators. Curiously, for-profits and nonprofits had similar costs. One cautionary note about the study: the authors fail to control for many factors that might influence their measures of quality, including MCO location and enrollment characteristics. Thus, the results are suggestive of quality differences but are far from conclusive.

There will undoubtedly be more studies of the role of the profit motive in medicine, particularly in MCOs. The popular image of MCOs is that they are investor-driven organizations out to make a quick buck at the expense of consumers. But this hardly describes the first managed care plans. On the contrary, these mainly nonprofit plans offered consumers a way to save money while keeping well. The next chapter examines the rise of managed care.

CHAPTER 2

The Origins of Managed Care

FOR MOST of the twentieth century, the traditional U.S. health economy had three defining features:

1. Patients relied on autonomous physicians to act as their agents.

2. Patients received complex care from independent, nonprofit hospitals.

3. Insurers did not intervene in medical decision making and reimbursed physicians, hospitals, and other providers on a fee-for-service basis.

These features helped patients solve the problems of determining what medical services to buy, where to buy them, and how to assure coordination of care. But there has always been one drawback—the resulting health economy is very expensive. Back in 1960, health care expenditures accounted for just 5.2 percent of the U.S. gross domestic product (GDP), and per capita spending on health care was just $149 annually (adjusted to 1997 dollars). Even so, Americans still spent 20 percent more per capita on health care than anyone else. (Canada was next at $123 annually, adjusted for exchange rate differences.) Costs continued to increase through the 1960s, to the point where health care accounted for 7.3 percent of the U.S. GDP in 1970, and per capita spending of $357 was 27 percent higher than anywhere else. Though spending more on health care, Americans did not appear to be healthier. Key health indicators such as life expectancy were no higher in the United States then in other developed nations. Health policy analysts began to wonder whether Americans were getting their money's worth. Despite the enormous trust that Americans placed in the traditional health care system, many analysts suspected that the system was inherently inefficient.

In research that emerged during the 1960s and 1970s, economists identify two sources of potentially massive inefficiency in the traditional health economy. First, insured patients demand any and all medical services regardless of cost, even those offering the slightest possible health benefit. Economists call such excessive demand *moral hazard*. Second, autonomous providers receiving fee-for-service payments have a financial incentive to recommend the costliest of treatments, even those that are of little value to patients. Economists call this *demand inducement*.

Moral hazard and demand inducement result from incentives facing patients and providers. They drive up costs, without commensurate increases in the quality of care. This chapter describes these incentive problems. It also describes the origins, growth, and eventual acceptance of HMOs, organizations that restructure the inherently inefficient incentives of the traditional health economy.

MORAL HAZARD

"Moral hazard" describes how people change their behavior when they have insurance. Moral hazard is not restricted to medical care, and it takes many forms. Consumers worry less about locking their cars when they have automobile theft insurance. Homeowners are more likely to build on floodplains when the federal government subsidizes flood insurance. Drivers go a bit faster when they have air bags (which "insure" against injury in the event of an accident). Patients purchase more medical services when health insurance foots the bill.

There is moral hazard in medical care because the demand curve for medical care is downward sloping; that is, price matters. When patients pay less out of their own pockets for medical care, they buy more of it. In the 1960s and 1970s, not everyone believed that the price of medical care mattered. Many people, including most health care providers, argued that demand was based entirely on medical need.

Eager to determine whether price mattered and to measure the extent of moral hazard, economists collected data on medical prices and utilization. Their research showed that individuals whose insurance required them to make copayments purchased fewer medical services than did individuals whose insurance covered the full cost of care.[1] This finding supports the contention the price matters, but it is not conclusive. It is possible that individuals who made copayments were healthier, on average, than those who did not, and that is why they purchased fewer services. If so, then price might not matter after all. This is an example of *selection bias*, which plagues intergroup comparisons whenever the individuals in one "study group" are systematically different from those in the other "study group." Selection bias may be at work in comparisons of individuals with full insurance and those who make copayments. Patients with few medical problems would probably be more willing to purchase insurance with copayments. This might explain their lower utilization. As we will see, selection bias hampers efforts to answer several other important questions about the importance of economic incentives in the health economy.

The RAND Study

The best way to eliminate selection bias in a research study is to conduct a randomized experiment.[2] Randomization assures that individuals in each study group have similar characteristics. To measure the effect of price on utilization, one could randomly assign some patients to an insurance plan with no copayments and others to a plan with copayments. Because of the randomization, any differences in demand would be the result of the copayments, not medical need. This is exactly what researchers at the RAND Corporation did in the National Health Insurance Experiment, better known as the RAND study.[3]

The RAND study was a by-product of the ill-fated Kennedy-Mills national health insurance plan. Proposed in the early 1970s, Kennedy-Mills would have replaced private indemnity health insurance with a single national indemnity insurance plan but otherwise preserve most aspects of the traditional health economy. The plan would reimburse providers on a fee-for-service basis and, to contain costs, would require patients to make copayments. As with every other national health insurance plan considered by Congress this century, Kennedy-Mills was introduced with much optimism for its eventual passage. But the plan faltered in Congress. The medical establishment objected to "socialized medicine," Republicans worried about budget ramifications, labor leaders wanted a more generous plan, and Wilbur Mills, one of the bill's sponsors and chairman of the House Ways and Means Committee, was found cavorting in the Washington, D.C., tidal basin with nightclub stripper Fanny Foxe.

Before the plan fell out of favor, considerable energy was spent trying to figure out how to make it work. At the time, there was no consensus about whether copayments would limit utilization or, if they did, how large the copayments should be. The RAND study would help answer these questions. Over six thousand individuals in six locations participated in the study, in which researchers randomly assigned participants to one of five insurance plans. The plans covered the same services and reimbursed providers for the full amounts they charged. The only differences among the plans were the copayments. In one plan, all medical care was free. In others, copayments ranged from 25 percent to 95 percent of the medical bill, up to a maximum annual out-of-pocket payment of roughly $1,000 per individual. The study lasted three to five years. In addition to studying demand, RAND researchers collected before-and-after data on health status.

Using sophisticated statistical techniques to control for nonprice factors (such as income) that might affect utilization, the RAND study generated widely accepted estimates of the magnitude of moral hazard. RAND researchers found that individuals who received free medical care incurred about 30 percent higher medical costs than did individuals who made copayments. Moreover, individuals receiving free care were not measurably healthier than those making copayments, even after five years, despite their higher levels of utilization.

The RAND study demonstrated that there is substantial moral hazard in medical care. Economists were not surprised; after all, moral hazard is merely the consequence of individuals acting in their own self-interest, and patients are not immune to selfishness. No one should expect patients to consider the cost of medical care when insurance is paying for it. Nor should one expect the additional services rendered to patients receiving free care to materially improve their health. After all, patients making small copayments felt they could do without those services. Unless these patients (and their physicians) made gross errors in judgment, the forgone services must have been of minimal value.

After the RAND results were published, insurers realized that copayments could eliminate excessive moral hazard utilization without eroding quality. They offered more plans with higher copayments and slightly lower premiums. Consumers (or at least their employers) eagerly accepted the new plans, and today a typical indemnity insurance plan requires enrollees to pay for 20 percent of medical costs and/or pay deductibles of $250 to $500 before coverage begins. Medical savings accounts (MSAs), which have been touted as a cost-effective alternative to managed care, rely even more heavily on deductibles. Patients must withdraw up to several thousand dollars annually from their private MSAs to pay for medical services before coverage begins.

HMOs generally require much lower copayments than do indemnity insurers; some do not require any copayments. Rather than limit the incentives of patients to demand services of marginal value, HMOs limit the incentives of providers to offer such services. HMOs reason that by focusing on provider incentives, they can simultaneously limit moral hazard *and* demand inducement.

DEMAND INDUCEMENT

Physicians are both diagnosticians (they tell patients what is wrong with their health) and clinicians (they fix what is wrong). This often puts them in the position of prescribing a treatment and getting paid to provide it. Ken Arrow wrote that "advice given by physicians as to further treatment by himself or others is supposed to be completely divorced from self-interest."[4] But physicians must certainly face great temptation to be selfish. After all, patients will consent to almost any treatment recommendation. They do not know enough to question their physicians' decisions, they trust their physicians to make the right decisions, and they fear the medical consequences if they do not consent. Patients are especially vulnerable in tertiary care situations such as cancer care and complex surgery, where technological complexity keeps them in the dark about what is and is not appropriate care, and the cost of refusing treatment may be life itself. In these circumstances, physicians could substantially boost their incomes by making treatment recommendations and other clinical decisions that are not in the best interests of their patients.

The idea that physicians might abuse their role as agents for financial gain is not new. In *The Social Transformation of American Medicine*, Paul Starr quotes an 1906 industry trade journal that encouraged physicians to use their power to gain leverage over hospitals: "If favorably disposed toward the hospital, the physician can very frequently recommend that a patient be transferred to the hospital even where the distinct need of this transfer does not exist."[5] If the image of Marcus Welby represents physicians at their most benevolent, the image of physicians exploiting patient ignorance to boost their incomes and power represents physicians at their greediest.

It may come as a surprise to physicians and their patients, but there is little doubt among academic economists, and virtually no doubt among other health services researchers, that physicians induce demand. Yet despite four decades of research, there remains little consensus about the magnitude of inducement. This is remarkable, because some of the most fundamental changes brought about by managed care, especially the widespread use of capitation, are direct responses to a perception of widespread inducement. Regulators have also taken steps to combat inducement. Legislators in several states have used inducement theory to justify placing restrictions on physician ownership of diagnostic testing equipment (the logic being that physicians who own testing equipment will order unnecessary tests to boost their incomes). The Health Care Finance Administration (HCFA) used inducement theory to justify capping reimbursements for surgical procedures following reductions in Medicare surgical fees. (They reasoned that surgeons facing lower fees would recommend more surgeries to make up for lost income.)

Theory and Evidence about Inducement

Economist Milton Roemer is widely credited with introducing the idea of demand inducement in a 1961 article in which he describes a curious "natural experiment" relating the supply of medical services to utilization.[6] In 1957, a community in upstate New York had one nonprofit general hospital with 139 beds. Although the hospital was old, it seemed to meet local needs. It had an average daily census of 108 patients, suggesting that it was rarely full. In 1958, the hospital moved into a new facility with 197 beds, and the daily census in the new hospital increased to 137 patients.

Roemer is hard-pressed to explain the increase. There seemed to be little change in the overall health of the community, and there were no major macroeconomic forces at work. Roemer is seemingly left with only one possible explanation: physicians responded to the increased supply of beds by admitting more patients. Roemer's finding led to the expression "a bed built is a bed filled" or, more accurately in light of his evidence, "a bed built is a bed half-filled." The notion that hospitals can keep their beds filled regardless of market conditions would seem ludicrous in today's managed care environment, what with hospital occupancy rates often hovering below 60 percent. But at the time of fee-for-service medicine, it raised quite a few eyebrows.[7]

Roemer does not spell out how he thought the hospital filled its beds, and he takes pains to point out that there was no evidence of inappropriate care. He even suggests that the local population may have received inadequate care prior to the opening of the new hospital, so that the additional utilization was beneficial to the community. As more research emerged in the 1970s, however, researchers and policy makers took a dimmer view of inducement. The prevailing sentiment was that inducement drives up medical costs, enriches providers at the expense of patients, and provides little or no health benefit.

Inducement theory rests on four key points. First, inducement arises because the indications for many medical interventions can be vague, so that a physician may be unable to decide which of several interventions best serves the patient's interest. Second, given such clinical ambiguity, physicians who are reimbursed on a fee-for-service basis might recommend the most costly intervention. Third, in extreme cases of inducement, physicians might even ignore unambiguous clinical indications to pursue financial goals. Fourth, to the extent that hospital managers (of for-profits and nonprofits) want to keep their beds filled, they have no reason to object to inducement. If inducement theory is true, then HMOs have a powerful justification for replacing fee-for-service reimbursement with capitation. But theory alone cannot determine whether the gray area of medicine is large or small, or whether physicians will act selfishly. To determine if inducement is a large or small problem, researchers must directly measure its magnitude.

During the 1970s and 1980s, economists published several empirical studies of inducement. Unfortunately, these studies were confusing, in part because they did not directly measure the effect of fee-for-service incentives, in part because they employed statistical methods that many found wanting. As a result, the studies did not convincingly determine whether inducement existed, let alone measure its magnitude.

To understand inducement research, it is helpful to distinguish between two forms of inducement. In *weak-form inducement*, physicians receiving fee-for-service payments induce demand and, consequently, overtreat their patients. This is just another way of saying that financial incentives matter, and it leads to the corollary that physicians receiving capitated payments or a fixed salary may undertreat their patients. In *strong-form inducement*, physicians receiving fee-for-service payments are more likely to induce demand when their incomes are threatened. Although the weak form is more germane to the debate about the relative merits of fee-for-service reimbursement and capitation, the initial research on inducement examines the strong form.

In a seminal paper, Victor Fuchs presents evidence of substantial strong-form inducement.[8] He shows that the demand for surgery was higher in regions that had more surgeons per capita and estimates that a 10 percent increase in the supply of surgeons would lead to a 3 percent increase in the demand for surgeries. Subsequent studies by other researchers, using better data than that available to Fuchs, reach similar, if slightly weaker, findings. The consensus was that a 10 percent increase in supply leads to about a 1 percent increase in demand. Thus, physicians appear to induce demand—presumably by recommending surgeries in the "gray area"—when their incomes are threatened by competition.

Not everyone was convinced by these findings because of a "chicken-or-egg" aspect to them. The data reveal that purchases of physicians' services were higher in those markets that had more physicians. But which way did causality run? Did physicians cause patients to purchase more medical care (as inducement theorists claim)? Or did communities whose residents had a high demand for medical services attract a disproportionate number of physicians to locate there? When causality is in doubt, statistical analyses can sometimes generate misleading conclusions.

Normally, when we observe a positive correlation between sales and the number of sellers, the direction of causality is unambiguous. For example, when we observe a positive correlation between the amount of new housing construction and the number of construction workers in a market, we automatically conclude that workers are attracted to high-demand markets—in other words, that demand causes supply. Inducement theorists embrace the reverse causality, in which supply causes demand.[9] Although Fuchs and others were aware of this causality dilemma, their statistical methods could not fully sort out cause and effect. This does not imply that inducement theory is wrong, but it does imply that there is more than one way to interpret the evidence.

More on the Causality Problem

The causality problem shows up in most efforts to assess the role of incentives in medical decision making. Consider, for example, several influential studies showing that physicians who own diagnostic testing equipment order more diagnostic tests.[10] Policy makers have assumed that causality runs from ownership to testing and have enacted laws restricting physician ownership of test equipment. But another interpretation of the data is possible. Perhaps physicians who tend to order a lot of tests under any circumstances are more inclined to purchase testing equipment. In other words, causality might run from testing to ownership. If this is the case, then banning ownership would not reduce testing and might even inconvenience patients.

A few recent studies of strong-form inducement seem immune to concerns about causality and lend support to inducement theory. Examining a long time series of data on childbirths, Jon Gruber and Maria Owings find a small, statistically significant relationship between the supply of obstetricians and the rate of cesarean sections.[11] Citing Gruber and Owings, Victor Fuchs, in his 1996 presidential address to the American Economic Association, states that, "despite many attempts to discredit it, the hypothesis that fee-for-service physicians can and do induce demand for their services is alive and well." A recent study by Winnie Yip lends further support. Studying physician responses to reductions in Medicare payments for open-heart surgery, Yip finds that surgical rates increased substantially after payment reductions.[12] It seems probable that most of the increase in surgical rates reflected demand inducement.[13] On the other hand, Jon Gruber, John Kim, and Dina Mayzlin find that cesarean section rates for Medicaid patients decreased when Medicaid payments for this procedure fell relative to payments for vaginal deliveries.[14] This is the opposite of what would be expected if there was strong-form inducement.

These recent studies suggest that incentives do affect physician decision making. But they do not provide a direct measure of how much utilization would change if payers switched from fee-for-service payments to capitation. This would require estimates of weak-form inducement. Research on weak-form inducement, which I discuss in Chapter 4, has only emerged in the past decade and is also confounded by causality issues. It is amazing to think that questions about the role of incentives remain unresolved. After all, it has been nearly a century since a handful of organizations challenged the orthodoxy of fee-for-service medicine. When managed care first came on the scene, the idea that capitation would change physician behavior was just a theory.

HMOs: THE CENTURY-LONG REVOLUTION

"Flat-of-the-Curve" Medicine

By the 1970s, many economists and health policy analysts believed that moral hazard and demand inducement were creating enormous waste in our health care system. In the late 1970s, Alain Enthoven, a professor at Stanford University, coined the expression "flat of the curve" medicine to describe this waste. Enthoven hypothesized that the overall health of a population gradually increases as it receives more health care services. Beyond some point, however, additional health services offer no benefit to patients and can even be harmful. This situation is depicted in Figure 2.1, which graphs health status against utilization of health services. The "flat of the curve" is the point at which services are of no additional value.

Enthoven argued that moral hazard and demand inducement placed the United States on the flat part of the curve.[15] A small but vocal group of policy analysts, led by Enthoven and Paul Ellwood, then executive director of the American Rehabilitation Institute, felt that the United States could not get off the flat of the curve if physicians received fee-for-service reimbursement. They encouraged the government, businesses, and provider organizations seeking to eliminate waste in the health economy to consider an old but relatively obscure form of organizing medical care that did away with fee-for-service medicine. What they had in mind was the precursor to today's HMOs.

The Origins of Managed Care

Paul Starr traces the origins of managed care back to the 1890s, when physicians agreed to provide prepaid medical care to "lodges"—fraternal orders, unions, and other associations of workers. These lodges already supplied members with social benefits such as life insurance, so paying for health care was a natural extension for them. Physicians provided lodge members unlimited free access to health care services in exchange for an annual fee of one to two dollars per member. Although lodges reached into nearly one-third of American families, prepaid medicine was largely concentrated among immigrant communities, and most physicians refused to participate.

Prepaid group practice began in the early twentieth century when groups such as the Western Clinic in Tacoma, Washington, offered to provide industrial medicine (medical care for work-related injuries and ill-

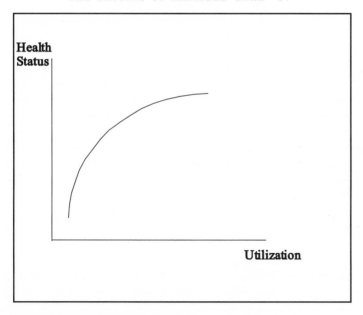

Figure 2.1 Flat-of-the-curve medicine.

nesses) to workers at a lumber mill for a prepaid monthly fee.[16] By 1920, two dozen clinics in Oregon and Washington offered similar prepayment arrangements to other employee groups. More ambitious prepayment programs soon emerged. In 1927, Dr. Michael Shadid sold shares in the construction of Community Hospital in Elk City, Oklahoma, in exchange for lifetime access to hospital care. Shadid's plan evolved, seven years later, into the Farmer's Union Cooperative Association. In 1929, Drs. Donald Ross and H. Clifford Loos established a clinic to serve the employees of the Los Angeles water and power departments. As with the clinics in Washington and Oregon, Ross-Loos provided all care for a fixed monthly payment.

Prepayment represented a form of health insurance—employees of participating firms did not have to pay additional fees when they received care. Another form of health insurance emerged during the 1930s, when the Great Depression put the cost of health care out of the reach of millions of Americans. Providers started the Blue Cross and Blue Shield insurance plans to make health care more affordable. The Blues pooled contributions from enrollees and paid providers on a fee-for-service basis. This served as a model for indemnity insurance that has survived to this day.

Both the prepayment and the Blue Cross and Blue Shield insurance plans protected patients from having to make large payments for medical care. Yet the mainstream medical community embraced the Blues and scorned the prepayment plans. The AMA fought to maintain fee-for-service reimbursement, objecting to the idea of "unlimited service for limited pay."[17] Doctors derided prepaid group practice as "contract medicine," and hospitals refused to admit prepaid group practice patients. Many county medical societies even refused membership to physicians who accepted prepayment. Physicians in prepaid groups had to go to court to win access to community hospitals. Despite the protests of mainstream medicine, a few physicians in scattered communities stood by their prepaid group practices. Prepayment had gained a foothold that it would not relinquish, and the foothold would strengthen with the emergence of the Kaiser Foundation health plans.

Kaiser

The precursors to the Kaiser Foundation health plans appeared in the 1930s, about the same time that the Blue Cross plans emerged. At that time, the Kaiser Industrial Organization owned dozens of firms, including many construction companies. A southern California physician named Sidney Garfield approached Henry Kaiser with an attractive offer. If Kaiser's business insurers would prepay Garfield five cents per day per employee, he would provide industrial medical care to Kaiser construction workers. For another five cents, he would provide nonindustrial care. After initial success with this program in Los Angeles, Garfield repeated it in the state of Washington, providing prepaid family medicine for Kaiser employees working on construction of the Grand Coulee Dam.

When World War II brought tens of thousands of workers to Kaiser's shipyards in northern California and Portland, Oregon, Kaiser created the blueprint for the first HMO. Kaiser built medical and hospital facilities for two hundred thousand employees and prepaid physicians to provide medical care in group practice settings. When the war ended, shipyard employment fell sharply. Kaiser opened its plan to the public, and the Kaiser Foundation Health Plan was born. (It was not called a health maintenance organization until 1970, when Paul Ellwood coined the term. By that time, Kaiser had over three million members in six different regional plans.)

The Kaiser Foundation Health Plan is, first and foremost, a health insurance company. Like other insurers such as Blue Cross, it offers to pay for an enrollee's medical expenses in exchange for an annual premium. Like other insurers, it compensates providers who care for its enrollees. But unlike other insurers, it secures all physician services under an exclu-

sive prepayment arrangement with a provider group, the regional Permanente Medical Group. Permanente, in turn, provides care exclusively for
Kaiser enrollees. Because of this bilateral arrangement, Permanente is
often considered to belong to Kaiser—hence the common reference to the
Kaiser-Permanente plan.

Kaiser was not the only major HMO to get its start in the 1940s. Under
the Health Insurance Plan (HIP) established in 1944, medical groups were
created throughout New York City to provide prepaid medical care to city
employees. In 1947, Dr. Shadid brought stories of his Elk City success to
a consumer cooperative in Seattle consisting of members of the Grange,
the Aero-Mechanics Unions, and local food and supply cooperatives. The
Group Health Cooperative of Puget Sound (GHC) convinced four hundred families to contribute $100 each toward the purchase of the Seattle
Medical Securities Clinic and a sixty-bed hospital. The GHC grew rapidly,
and had over two hundred thousand enrollees by the 1970s. During this
time, physicians and consumer cooperatives established prepaid group
practices throughout the nation. By 1970, there were roughly thirty to
forty prepaid group practices, while several dozen other "traditional"
groups offered a prepayment plan to at least some of their patients. Prepaid group practice was hardly dominant, but it had enough of a presence
for the health care community to take notice.

The original prepaid group practices had much in common. Most were
founded by physicians and served local consumer cooperatives (the descendants of lodges). The physicians established them as nonprofits; many
physicians seemed to be more interested in pursuing their vision for reor-
ganizing medical care than they were in boosting their incomes. This is
consistent with Arrow's view of medicine as a calling, although Starr observes that the AMA did not completely disapprove of the profit motive in
medicine—it only objected when nonphysicians reaped the profits.[18] The
prepaid group practices targeted workers, especially those who lacked
steady, reliable incomes. Perhaps the most important common feature was
prepayment.

Prepayment and Cost Containment

It is not clear whether the physicians who pioneered the prepaid group
practice movement were concerned about incentive issues. By the 1960s
and 1970s, however, HMO supporters were touting the efficiency benefits
of prepayment. In 1971, Dr. Cecil Cutting, the executive director of the
Kaiser-Permanente Medical Group in northern California, wrote that the
"direct relationship of prepayment to providers becomes an incentive for

the physician to develop economies in spending the medical dollar while maintaining quality."[19] A 1971 report published by the Henry J. Kaiser Foundation touted "the absence of a fee-for-service incentive to do what, by judicious surgical standards, constitutes unjustified surgery."[20] Today, patients worry about HMOs providing too little care. Thirty years ago, HMO supporters claimed that fee-for-service medicine led to too much care.

Besides prepayment, HMOs used other strategies to constrain health care costs. Kaiser and the GHC owned their own hospitals, thereby eliminating the conflict that exists in the traditional health economy between hospital administrators who want to keep their beds filled and insurers who want to reduce utilization. This may explain why lengths of stay at Kaiser and GHC hospitals were 25 percent shorter than at other hospitals. In addition, Kaiser hospitals offered and promoted a wide array of outpatient services. For example, in 1969 the ratio of outpatient visits (including visits to physicians' offices) to hospital admissions for Kaiser was 50 percent higher than for the United States as a whole. In the 1960s, Kaiser and GHC hospitals were among the first in the nation to offer home nursing services as a substitute for lengthy hospitalizations. Through the 1970s and 1980s, Kaiser and GHC continued to emphasize outpatient care, becoming among the first institutions to offer freestanding surgery and emergency care facilities.

HMO supporters also touted their emphasis on prevention.[21] One of the founders of the GHC, Dr. Sandy MacColl, wrote that he and his colleagues sought "a system of family care . . . directed towards a goal of good care, health maintenance, and preventive services."[22] Paul Ellwood came up with the name "health maintenance organization" because he believed that prepayment rewarded providers who kept their patients healthy. Kaiser's Dr. Cutting called this "the reversal of economics," stating that, with prepayment, "both the hospitals and doctors are better off if the patient remains well."[23] This remains the conventional wisdom among most health care professionals.

The conventional wisdom contains a hidden assumption: namely, that providers in the traditional health economy do not want to keep their patients well. It is certainly true that providers have a financial incentive not to heal their patients, at least in the short run. If their patients are not well, providers can bill for additional medical services. But this implies a pernicious market failure in the long run. Somehow, providers who do not take care of their patients manage to hold on to their practices. It is difficult to believe that the payment mechanism is a dominant factor when providers make decisions that might affect the long-term health of their patients. But there is no systematic evidence to either confirm or refute the argument.

HMOs as Agents

In the traditional health economy, insurers left physicians alone to make decisions on behalf of their patients. For better or for worse, HMOs tried to influence these decisions, and, in doing so, became agents in their own right. Through a combination of incentives and exhortation, they encouraged physicians to treat patients in outpatient facilities and shorten inpatient lengths of stay by discharging patients to the care of home health nurses. (Similar changes would occur within Medicare in the 1980s.) Perhaps more controversially, HMOs used financial incentives—effectively, denial of coverage—to steer patients to selected specialists and hospitals.

A common criticism of HMOs is that this steering restricts patient choice, but I believe this criticism is misplaced. The conventional wisdom may be that patients in the traditional health economy get to choose their physicians and their hospital. But outside of selecting their PCP, they rarely do. Instead, their PCP makes the choices for them. It is not obvious whether a PCP makes better choices than does Kaiser, the Group Health Cooperative, or any other HMO, and there is some evidence that PCP referrals leave much to be desired. In a dissertation written in the 1970s, sociologist Stephen Shortell finds that physician referral patterns were heavily based on factors such as status and economics, rather than medical need and physician quality.[24] A recent study by Arthur Hartz, Jose Pulido, and Evelyn Kuhn finds that the reputations of cardiac surgeons among physicians in their local communities are uncorrelated with objective measures of their ability.[25] Another recent study by Peter Franks et al. finds that PCPs in Rochester, New York, had vastly different referral rates that could not be explained by differences in patient needs.[26]

While independent physicians have not always rationalized their referral decisions, the early HMOs prided themselves on the selectivity of their networks. Kaiser described physician recruitment as a "continuous talent hunt" and boasted of both the technical competency and the communication skills of its physicians.[27] For example, one Kaiser report stated: "To the trained observer, Permanente physicians-in-chief are indistinguishable from the divisional and departmental chiefs to be found in the clinical faculties of medical schools, except that they appear further advanced in their understanding and appreciation of community medical care organization."[28] Such self-promotion is no guarantee that Kaiser really recruited the best physicians. But there is no reason to believe that the physicians in Kaiser's "restrictive" network were inferior to those in the typical PCP's referral network.

Could HMOs Be Trusted?

Whether enrolled in a traditional health care plan or an HMO, patients have relied on others to solve their shopping problems. Mechanic observes that the physician in the traditional health economy is loyal to the patient (demand inducement notwithstanding); this is why patients readily trust their physicians. But physicians employed by HMOs might have divided loyalties. On the one hand, they are driven by training and professionalism to always act in the best interests of their patients. On the other hand, they are driven by financial incentives to watch the bottom line. HMO enrollees had to trust their plans to employ good, caring physicians; they also had to trust that their HMO physicians economized by emphasizing prevention and by eliminating waste, not by withholding necessary services. Despite the fact that most early HMOs were nonprofit, many health care professionals, especially providers anxious to defend the traditional health economy, questioned whether this trust was well placed. After all, key decisions rested in the hands of managers and not just physicians. Would HMO physicians remain staunch advocates for their patients? To whom would the managers be loyal? Would the "reversal of economics" lead to lower quality? As MCOs have gained market share, and for-profit MCOs have come to outnumber the nonprofits, these questions have grown in importance. The answers, which I discuss in Chapter 4, have only recently begun to emerge. In a nutshell, the research finds that the quality of care received by patients in HMOs is no worse, on average, than the quality received by patients with traditional indemnity insurance.

In the 1970s, skeptics not only challenged the wisdom of patients who entrusted their health to HMOs but also wondered if HMOs actually saved any money. By the late 1970s, evidence on how HMOs achieved their savings began to emerge. While the evidence seemed to answer a few of the skeptics' questions, the research methods were far from compelling, and doubts about the magnitude of HMO cost savings lingered.

EVIDENCE ON THE EARLY HMOS

HMOs grew slowly through the 1960s and 1970s. It was easy for academic researchers to dismiss them as a strictly "West Coast phenomenon," and, as a result, academics were largely indifferent to their performance. That changed in 1978, when the *New England Journal of Medicine* published a special article by Harold Luft called "How Do Health Maintenance Organizations Achieve Their 'Savings'?"[29] Luft presents "virtually all the evidence of the last 25 years concerning HMO 'savings' . . . and examine(s) various explanations of how such 'savings' are achieved."[30] He finds only five papers that compared the total medical costs for HMO and non-HMO enrollees. All five studies examined Kaiser, three also examined the Ross-Loos prepaid group practice, and only one looked at additional HMOs outside of California. These studies found that, on average, yearly expenses for enrollees in traditional Blue Cross indemnity plans were 50 percent higher than for Kaiser enrollees. Yearly expenses for enrollees in other indemnity plans were about 21 percent higher than for Kaiser enrollees. Expenses for Ross-Loos subscribers fell between those for Kaiser and indemnity plans.

Luft looks at research that might explain the cost differences, finding fifty-one studies comparing hospital utilization of HMO and indemnity enrollees. The vast majority of these studies (forty-one out of fifty-one) found that HMO enrollees had substantially fewer hospital admissions and shorter lengths of stay. Other studies found that HMO enrollees had similar or higher levels of outpatient utilization.

Luft offers an appealing interpretation of the data: HMOs save money by substituting outpatient care for inpatient care and/or eliminating unnecessary hospitalizations. But Luft suggests two other possible interpretations of the data. HMOs might save money by undertreating their patients, sacrificing quality to save money. Or HMO patients may be healthier than other patients, and therefore do not need to be hospitalized as often. The latter explanation, another example of selection bias, seems plausible. Severely ill patients may be reluctant to enroll in health plans that are reputed to limit utilization. If this is the case, then HMOs might not really reduce costs, despite the apparent cost savings. Selection bias continues to confound many efforts to accurately compare HMO costs with costs of indemnity insurance. However, a recent series of studies that are immune to selection bias confirm that HMOs really do lower costs. I will discuss this research in Chapter 4.

Because of its experimental design, the RAND study offered an opportunity to overcome selection bias in evaluation of HMO costs. One of the study sites was Seattle, home of the GHC of Puget Sound. In addition to randomly assigning Seattle study participants to indemnity plans, RAND randomly assigned several hundred to the GHC. RAND researchers find that the overall expenditures of the group assigned to the GHC were comparable to those of individuals assigned to indemnity plans with high copayments, and about 30 percent lower than those of individuals assigned to the indemnity plan with no copayments. Most of the cost difference between GHC and free care was attributed to differences in hospital expenditures.[31] The RAND study of the GHC has been generally regarded as the best evidence that HMOs reduce costs. But a disproportionately large percentage of the study population selected for the GHC refused to enroll, making it difficult to be certain that this "randomized" trial was free from selection bias.

Despite the reservations about selection bias, the Luft and RAND studies lent credence to the claim that HMOs offered a solution to some of the inefficiencies of the traditional health economy. But as health care costs continued to soar, most health care professionals and policy analysts ignored HMOs and instead turned to the government for solutions.

CHAPTER 3

The Government Steps In

IT IS NOT too far-fetched to describe the pre-1960s U.S. health economy as "laissez-faire." Of course, there were licensing laws establishing minimum standards of competence for providers. Otherwise, most government programs increased insurance coverage and access to services but did not directly intervene in the market. The absence of direct intervention is somewhat surprising. During the middle third of the century, the prevailing sentiment in the United States was that "big government" could solve most social and economic problems. The federal government heavily regulated airlines, banking, telecommunications, and many other industries, but not health care. Yet most Americans considered (as they still do) health care to be more important than virtually all other goods and services. Moreover, there was a growing consensus that health care markets did not behave like "normal" markets. Citing "importance" and "market failure," many policy analysts called for new regulations to make the health economy work better.[1]

Without doubt, the traditional health economy did not behave according to textbook treatments of supply and demand. In the textbook model, the unfettered interactions of buyers and sellers lead to efficient production and consumption. But the laissez-faire health economy hardly seemed to be efficient. Moral hazard and demand inducement drove up costs without commensurate gains in quality. During the 1970s, Alain Enthoven, Harold Luft, Burton Weisbrod, and others identified another inefficiency, stemming from a complex interaction among new medical technology, cost-based reimbursement, and a pernicious form of competition that would be dubbed the "medical arms race."

RISING COSTS AND MEDICAL TECHNOLOGY

Of all the factors that contribute to rising health care costs, economists have singled out technological change as the biggest culprit. This may seem surprising because in many other industries, such as telecommunications and computers, technological improvements usually reduce costs. Some of the new medical technologies that emerged in the 1960s and 1970s included kidney dialysis, open-heart surgery, organ transplants, and computerized tomography (CT) scans. These innovations improved the nation's health immeasurably, but they were extremely expensive, adding billions of dollars to the health economy.

One wonders why new medical technologies rarely seem to reduce costs. In describing what he calls the "health care quadrilemma," Burton Weisbrod offers an explanation.[2] He describes the quadrilemma as a complex interaction among insurance, cost, quality, and technology. He explains that firms that develop medical technology respond to incentives, just like any other firms. These firms know that in the traditional health economy, in which fully insured patients delegate medical decision making to providers, cost is usually not an issue. This allows medical R&D firms to concentrate on technologies that improve quality, without regard to cost. This is exactly what they did.

Weisbrod scrutinized two particular aspects of the traditional health economy: moral hazard that results from indemnity insurance, and cost-based reimbursement for hospital care. We have already seen how indemnity insurance encourages patients to purchase costly services almost without regard to medical need. But if there was any doubt that providers would be reimbursed for the cost of new technologies, it was eliminated by the growth of *cost-based reimbursement.*

The Blue Cross plans were among the first to pay hospitals for their costs of providing care (plus a small profit margin), rather than pay what they charged. The Blues reasoned that because insured patients would not care what hospitals charged, hospitals could set their prices substantially higher than their costs. The Blues hoped to limit their hospital payments by paying only for "reasonable" costs, plus a small profit margin. (The definition of "reasonable" has always been subjective.) For a while after their introduction in 1965, Medicare and Medicaid also paid hospitals for the cost of care. Cost-based reimbursement effectively guaranteed that hospitals would be profitable, as long as their costs were not excessive. This may have limited payments in the short run, but it created perverse incentives in the long run. Over time, hospitals could acquire equipment, boost staffing levels, introduce the latest technologies, and offer new treatments, knowing that their reimbursements would increase to cover the costs. Cost-based reimbursement also meant that inefficient hospitals would receive higher reimbursements than efficient ones. Conversely, hospitals that took pains to become more efficient saw their reimbursements fall. Hospitals even employed accountants to "cook the books" so as to maximize reimbursements.

The Medical Arms Race

Indemnity insurance and cost-based reimbursement assured the proliferation of costly medical technology. By the end of the 1970s, the United

States had many more CT scans, neonatology units, open-heart surgery suites, and other costly technologies than any other nation (on a per capita basis). Some economists suggested that technology proliferation was exacerbated by a "medical arms race" (MAR), in which hospitals competed for physicians and their patients by providing the latest in medical technology and the most generous staffing. The result, of course, was higher costs.

Anecdotal examples of the MAR abounded. When I was a doctoral student at Stanford, my adviser, Alain Enthoven, spoke of the proliferation of open-heart surgery facilities in California. (A good example: of five hospitals in Santa Barbara, three performed open-heart surgery.) The Health Care Finance Administration (HCFA) stated that every hospital seemed to want its own MRI. Concerned about a local MAR, Jack Finn, the director of the New Orleans Metropolitan Hospital Council, summed up many people's feelings this way: "When you get hospital competition in a city it drives costs up, not down. The competition is for doctors, not patients. And if you're going to compete for doctors, you have to have state-of-the-art equipment."[3]

In a 1985 publication, economists James Robinson and Harold Luft provide the first systematic evidence of the MAR.[4] They find that in the 1970s, hospitals with more competitors had higher costs of care, higher staffing levels, and more high-tech medical equipment. This highly influential study caused many to question the wisdom of pro-competitive health care strategies.

The MAR may have harmed quality. Many researchers, most notably Harold Luft and his colleagues at the University of California, have documented a "volume-outcome relationship" in medicine. That is, hospitals and surgeons with the most experience performing a specific procedure or treating a particular disease usually have among the lowest mortality rates; those with the least experience usually have among the highest mortality rates.[5] These researchers attribute at least some of this relationship to a learning curve.[6] Because the MAR spreads a given number of procedures across more hospitals, each hospital does not move as far down the learning curve as it would if there were less proliferation of technology. The troubling conclusion is that mortality rates might increase as a result.[7]

Moral hazard, demand inducement, and technological change all contributed to the high and rising costs of medical care in the United States through the 1970s. Other factors were at work as well. Personnel shortages, including a particularly severe nursing shortage, drove up labor costs. The population was gradually aging. Epidemiological trends, such as an increase in the incidence of cancer and an increase in the number of low-birth-weight babies, also contributed to cost increases. Higher costs alarmed insurers, who had to directly foot the bill. But private insurers were not the first to intervene to cut costs. Instead, it was the public insurers, Medicare and Medicaid, that took the first aggressive steps toward cost containment.

MEDICARE AND MEDICAID

Prior to 1950, there was little demand for health insurance in the United States—private health insurance paid for only around 10 percent of all medical costs. Patients were not overly concerned about having the financial wherewithal to obtain medical care, largely because medical care at that time emphasized caring rather than curing. During the 1950s, major advances in antibiotics and anesthetics greatly reduced surgical mortality rates. The demand for hospital care grew rapidly, as did the demand for insurance to help pay the hospital bills. Legislation (dating from World War II) exempting health insurance benefits from federal income taxation further fueled the demand for private health insurance. By 1960, the majority of working adults had private insurance that paid for hospital costs, and private insurance paid for over 21 percent of all medical costs.

The vast majority of the elderly and the poor, however, still lacked health insurance. In 1960, the federal government created the Kerr-Mills program to subsidize health care services for the elderly poor. Each state designed and administered its own version of the program, and the federal government paid up to 80 percent of the costs. Despite substantial federal cost sharing, most states had modest programs; in some states, Kerr-Mills subsidies amounted to less than one dollar per capita.[8] By the mid-1960s, the federal government was seeking to expand the Kerr-Mills program. At the same time, there were renewed calls for a program to cover all the elderly and the nonelderly poor.

A centerpiece of Lyndon Johnson's Great Society programs, the Social Security Amendments of 1965 created the Medicare and Medicaid programs. Medicare, which is administered by the federal Health Care Finance Administration (HCFA) and funded through national payroll taxes, covers hospital services and many outpatient services for the nation's elderly and disabled. The Medicare program provides health insurance for over 99 percent of elderly Americans, and HCFA is the largest single purchaser of health care in the United States. Through the Medicare program, HCFA pays for roughly one-third of all hospital care and about 20 percent of all physician services.

Medicaid, which is administered separately by each state according to HCFA guidelines, and jointly funded by the federal and state governments, covers a broad array of services for the "categorically" needy (individuals who fall into categories such as the disabled, families with dependent children, the blind, and the aged). Under Medicaid, states must cover a basic set of medical services, including hospital, physician, and nursing home care, and may add additional services, such as prescription drugs. In most states, Medicaid is the second- or third-largest purchaser of hospital and physician services (after Medicare and, possibly, the local Blue Cross plan). Medicaid is often the largest purchaser of services from inner-city health care providers and from nursing homes.

From their inception, the Medicare and Medicaid programs enjoyed rapid growth. Combined Medicare and Medicaid spending reached almost $14 billion in 1971, nearly double the amount spent in 1967, and program expenditures doubled again by 1976. Spurred on by Medicare and Medicaid, overall health care costs experienced annual double-digit growth for more than a decade. Health care costs, which accounted for 6.2 percent of GDP in 1966, rose to 7.6 percent in 1971 and 8.5 percent in 1976.

Rising health care costs troubled many employers, most of whom responded by raising their prices, curtailing wage increases, or both. Few employers dropped coverage or switched their employees into HMOs. Because their competitors did the same, all firms competed on a level playing field. They all bit the bullet together. Legislators were more alarmed. They had to either raise taxes or cut other social programs to pay for Medicare and Medicaid. Fearful of the consequences, federal and state legislators were the first to try to stem the tide of rising medical costs. They used the purchasing clout afforded by Medicare and Medicaid to try to rein in the health economy.

RATE SETTING

In the early 1970s, several states with large indigent populations grappled with the problem of rapidly increasing Medicaid expenditures. They targeted hospitals because hospital costs were the single biggest component of Medicaid. By this time, it was widely recognized that cost-based reimbursement encouraged hospital cost inflation, so the states looked for a different approach to paying for hospital services. Beginning with New York, the "rate-setting" states adopted a regulatory model, based on price caps, that they had used to control the price of electric and gas utilities. It was no surprise that New York—which was burdened with the nation's largest Medicaid program and a commensurate tax burden to pay for it—was first. State legislators proposed replacing Medicaid's open-ended cost-based reimbursement system with a plan to cap hospital payments at more tolerable levels. Private insurers, concerned that hospitals would respond to cutbacks in Medicaid payments by cost-shifting, asked to be included in a comprehensive payment system. In 1970, with the support of the insurance industry, New York introduced the first all-payer, prospective payment, rate-setting system.

Under New York's rate-setting system, all insurers (including Medicaid, Medicare, and private insurers) paid hospitals a flat fee for each patient day. The state set the fee at the beginning of the year, so hospitals knew how much they would receive in advance of treatment (hence the term "prospective payment"). To be fair to hospitals, the state set the fee approximately equal to the average daily cost of care across all hospitals, with regional adjustments to account for higher costs in New York City. This system put hospitals at "financial risk." Those with high costs stood to lose money, while those with low costs could prosper. Within five years of the introduction of New York's program, seven other states with similar concerns about Medicaid costs enacted their own rate-setting programs.[9]

While there were many differences among the programs, they all contained incentives for hospitals to reduce costs. Unlike cost-based reimbursement, which rewarded hospitals that added staff and services, rate setting rewarded hospitals that increased their efficiency. The hope was that if hospitals reduced their costs, the states could reduce their payments (or at least reduce the rate of growth of payments) without imposing an undue financial burden. Several studies conducted in the 1970s and early 1980s showed that these plans did slightly reduce the rate of growth of hospital costs.[10] My own research, for example, found that through the early 1980s, the annual rate of growth of hospital expenditures was about 1.5 percent lower in the rate-setting states than in the non-rate-setting states.[11] Though modest, these reductions caught the attention of HCFA. Seeking to control hospital costs in the Medicare program, HCFA developed its own rate-setting program.

The Medicare Prospective Payment System

In the late 1970s, HCFA authorized New Jersey to implement a rate-setting plan that paid each hospital a fixed fee per admission. To be fair to hospitals that handled more difficult cases, HCFA varied the fee according to the patient's medical condition and treatment. Thus, hospitals would receive more for performing open-heart surgery than they would for doing a simple appendectomy. HCFA used a scheme developed at Yale University to categorize conditions and treatments into roughly 470 "diagnosis-related groups," or DRGs.

After a short trial run in New Jersey, HCFA unveiled its Medicare Prospective Payment System (PPS) in 1983. The PPS, which remains one of the most significant regulatory programs in the health economy, places each hospital at financial risk for the cost of treating Medicare patients. Hospitals responded immediately to the change in incentives. Between 1982–83 (the last full fiscal year before PPS) and 1984–85 (the first full fiscal year after its introduction), the annual number of Medicare hospital stays declined from 10.3 million to 9.9 million, and the average Medicare length of stay declined from 10.3 to 9.3 days. Overall hospital cost inflation, which was running at 13 percent annually prior to 1983, dropped to 8 percent afterward.

Medicare's PPS reversed the incentives of cost-based reimbursement. HCFA expected that the PPS would encourage hospitals to find efficient ways to deliver care. After all, hospitals that hired more staff or added more equipment and services without a commensurate increase in patient volume were no longer guaranteed additional reimbursement. But under PPS the converse also applied—hospitals could prosper by cutting back on staffing, equipment, and services without commensurate reductions in volume. Unless the health economy was on Enthoven's "flat of the curve," these cutbacks might jeopardize quality. Critics of the PPS coined a phrase to characterize the patients who were hurriedly sent home by budget-conscious hospitals: they were discharged "quicker but sicker." Although critics used this term to disparage the PPS, at least one study found that the complaint was overstated; those physicians who did accelerate discharge tended to have considerable experience with early discharges already and probably did not place their patients in danger.[12]

While there is little direct evidence that the Medicare PPS has harmed quality thus far, there is evidence that stingy Medicaid payments may have done so. In an article published in the *New England Journal of Medicine*, Elliot Sussman and Ken Langa find that hospitals in California limited access to valuable cardiac revascularization services for Medicaid patients after the state reduced its Medicaid payments in 1983.[13] My own research with William White finds evidence of broader reductions in service levels following the California Medicaid cutbacks.[14]

Low Medicaid payments may also affect access. My study found that California's Medicaid cutbacks caused many hospitals to close, and those that remained open may have tried to shift their case mix away from Medicaid patients and toward privately insured patients. It is widely accepted that low payments also affect access to physicians. In a 1991 study, Anne Schwartz, David Colby, and Anne Reisinger document substantial interstate variation in Medicaid physician payments, reporting that "Medicaid beneficiaries in different states may face different degrees of access to medical care simply because of where they reside."[15] Things might not be so dire for Medicare—at least not yet. Even under PPS, Medicare payments are usually much higher than Medicaid payments. Thus, hospitals may still have the resources they need to provide high-quality care to Medicare patients, as well as the economic incentive to continue to do so. If Medicare payments continue to fall, however, the ability and incentives for hospitals to maintain quality and admit Medicare patients will almost surely decline.

PPS Perversities

PPS has created other undesirable incentives. To maximize reimbursements, hospitals attempt to classify patients into the most highly remunerative DRG that is consistent with the symptoms and treatment. This practice, called "upcoding" or "DRG creep," is discussed further in Chapter 5. Some hospitals transfer patients whose costs are expected to exceed the HCFA payment for their DRG, a practice that is derisively called "dumping." The opposite practice, in which hospitals treat only profitable patients, is called "cream skimming." Through both dumping and cream skimming, physician admission decisions based on medical need are replaced by hospital management admission decisions based on economics. In another practice driven by economics rather than medicine, hospitals sometimes "unbundle" hospital stays. Services that would normally be included as part of a single inpatient stay are provided, on an outpatient basis, before or after the hospitalization. As a result, HCFA pays the hospitals a flat fee for the hospital stay and then makes additional payments for outpatient services. The patient ends up making more visits to the provider, with no obvious health benefit. HCFA was aware of many of these perverse incentives when it introduced the PPS. To police the PPS, HCFA created peer review organizations (PROs), which are the direct descendants of earlier planning bodies called professional standards review organizations (PSROs). I will describe these planning efforts later.

After nearly two decades and at least one aborted attempt to expand the program to include some outpatient care, the PPS remains focused on inpatient services. With the exception of Medicare managed care, HCFA continues to provide either fee-for-service or cost-based reimbursement for virtually all other medical services. Most critically, it continues to pay physicians on a fee-for-service basis. Prior to 1993, HCFA paid physicians according to a complex fee schedule based on a number of factors, including prevailing fees in the community. In 1993, HCFA introduced a new pricing schedule for physicians, the Resource-Based Relative Value Scale (RBRVS). While lowering the fees for some specialty care and raising the fees for some primary care, the RBRVS remains a fee-for-service system. HCFA also makes fee-for-service payments for home health care, extended care facilities, and outpatient services.

HCFA data show how the contrasting incentives facing hospitals and other providers affect costs. From 1985 to 1997, Medicare spending for hospital services rose at an annual rate of 8 percent. All other Medicare spending rose at an annual rate of over 12 percent. These different growth rates not only reflect the difference in incentives but also suggest that there has been substitution of outpatient care for inpatient care. Unfortunately, this substitution has failed to hold down total costs—overall Medicare spending between 1985 and 1997 rose at an annual rate of 9.5 percent. For the period 1990–97, the annual rate of increase was even higher, at 9.8 percent. (In contrast, private sector spending grew at an annual rate of 7.3 percent over 1985–97 and just 5 percent over 1990–97.[16]) Medicare spending growth has slowed since 1997 due to a combination of factors, including reduced provider payments and increased enrollments in HMOs.

BIG PLANS, LITTLE EFFECTS

States adopted their rate-setting programs in the early 1970s against the backdrop of a great national health insurance debate. Faced with rapidly increasing health care costs and evidence that millions of Americans still lacked health insurance despite Medicare and Medicaid, many legislators sought to nationalize the health economy. Previously I described Senator Ted Kennedy and Representative Wilbur Mills's national insurance proposal. President Nixon had an alternative plan, based on the apparent success of prepaid health plans such as Kaiser. Nixon proposed to subsidize the growth of HMOs and encourage all Americans to enroll in them. When both proposals failed to garner enough votes for passage, Congress still faced pressure to rein in the health economy, and in the mid-1970s it firmly embraced health planning.

These were halcyon days for health planners, who believed that by controlling supply and demand, the government could generate an efficient and equitable health care marketplace. Planning is deceptively simple. Planners estimate the number of health care services that patients will "need," compare this with the number currently available, and compute the difference. If need exceeds availability, there is a "shortage"; if availability exceeds need, there is a "surplus." Appropriate legislation, such as subsidies to encourage entry, brings supply back in line with need.

Health planning began in earnest in 1946, with the Hill-Burton program to expand the nation's bed supply. Hill-Burton grew out of a general consensus that with the end of World War II, the demand for medical services would soon outstrip supply. Hill-Burton planners used a very simple method to determine need: they asked industry experts. Based on these opinions, planners determined that every region in the United States needed 4.5 hospital beds per 1,000 population. Hill-Burton funds were targeted toward those regions with the most serious shortages, that is, where the actual bed supply was substantially less than what was needed. After Hill-Burton, planners used increasingly sophisticated models. Nowadays, they examine demographic and epidemiological data to forecast the incidence of illness up to twenty years into the future.[17] Using productivity data (e.g., data on how many patients a provider can treat in a day), they determine the facilities and manpower needed to treat these illnesses. They forecast facilities and manpower availability based on entry and exit trends. Comparing forecasts with needs, planners identify shortages and surpluses.

Most economists flatly reject government intervention based on planning. They argue that shortages and surpluses are usually self-correcting and rarely require attention from the government. If a shortage should occur, perhaps because sellers fail to anticipate demand, prices would increase. Seeing higher prices, sellers would boost output. At the same time, consumers would buy less. If a surplus should occur, prices would fall, sellers would reduce output, and consumers would buy more. Thus, shortages and surpluses disappear through market forces. Health care planners usually ignore market forces—with consequences that can be catastrophic, as evidenced by the history of manpower planning.

The Wrong Number of Doctors

Planners in the late 1950s and early 1960s forecast that the United States would soon experience a dire shortage of physicians. A 1965 report to the Association of American Medical Colleges even claimed that it was "not likely that America will ever be able to produce all the physicians that the nation would like to have."[18] As a result of reports such as these, the federal and state governments poured several billion dollars into programs to increase enrollments in medical schools. At the same time, the federal government eased restrictions on immigration and licensure by graduates of overseas medical schools.

By all accounts, the programs worked too well. By 1980, the Graduate Medical Education National Advisory Council reported that there was a growing *surplus* of physicians.[19] To this day, the ranks of physicians in the United States continue to swell. How did the nation go from an apparent shortage to an apparent surplus in just fifteen years? Planners had ignored the market. There may have been an impending shortage of medical manpower in 1960, but the market responded. As with other shortages, the M.D. shortage drove up prices. (In this case, the prices were physician fees.) Monica Noether reports that the financial returns to becoming a physician increased dramatically in the 1960s, causing a 30 percent increase in medical school applications.[20] Although there is no way to know for sure, it seems likely that even without government subsidies, new medical schools would have opened, and existing schools would have expanded. The subsidies simply added to forces already at work in the market.

Are there now too many doctors? With the current mix of subsidies for medical education, entry barriers such as immigration quotas, and specialty group controls on training, it is impossible to know how many physicians there would be in a free market. The point is not whether we have too many or too few physicians, but that the market always acts independently of planners. Time and again, planners fail to take this into account.

Facilities Planning

At the time of Hill-Burton, there was little concern that moral hazard, demand inducement, and technological change might enable hospitals to continually expand, driving up costs in the process. When the federal government subsidized increases in the supply of physicians, it again ignored the potential impact on costs. But as states started to cope with rising costs, they realized that planning was not just a tool for expanding supply. Planning, especially when targeted at burgeoning health care facilities such as hospitals, might be a useful tool for cost containment.

As with rate setting, facilities planning began in New York State. Starting in 1964, New York required all hospitals to obtain approval for expansion or new construction from a government-appointed council. When reviewing applications, the council considered medical need and the availability of alternative providers. The state could withhold medical payments and/or revoke the license of any hospital that grew without council approval. By 1972, five other states had passed similar laws, which collectively became known as "certificate-of-need" (CON) laws.

About this time, the federal government was trying to expand facilities planning nationwide.[21] The 1966 Comprehensive Health Planning (CHP) Act encouraged state and local agencies to develop plans to limit overbuilding and duplication of services. But the act was ineffective and gave planners little real authority. In the Social Security Amendments of 1972, Congress required states to review hospital construction and expansion as a condition for receiving Medicare and Medicaid funds. This was no more effective than the CHP Act. Hospital costs continued to increase.

The 1974 National Health Planning and Resources Development Act (PL 93-641) added much-needed teeth to facilities planning. It replaced all previous facilities planning legislation and created over two hundred Health Services Areas. Overseeing health planning in each area was a Health Systems Agency (HSA) consisting of representatives of local provider, purchaser, and business organizations. Using methods similar to those used for manpower planning, HSAs established targets for efficient utilization in their Health Services Area, such as a limit of four hospital beds per 1,000 population or a minimum of 150 open-heart surgeries per facility. The HSAs performed CON review of all facilities expansion, modernization, and capital acquisition in excess of $150,000 and could deny CON applications that might cause the Health Services Area to miss its targets. HCFA would then deny Medicare and Medicaid reimbursements to facilities that expanded without CON approval.

Planners had high hopes for PL 93-641. Historians Anne Somers and Herman Somers stated that it provided "the first serious possibility for a comprehensive approach to the entire 'national health care system.' "[22] By tying the power of the purse (through CON review) to comprehensive local facilities planning, planners hoped that the health care marketplace would finally have the "right" number of facilities offering the "right" mix of services. It did not take long, however, for most observers to conclude that PL 93-641 was not working.

Research has found that CON requirements might have slightly limited bed growth but otherwise had little or no impact on the health economy.[23] In a recent review of the literature on CON, Michael Morrisey concludes that "rather than controlling costs, if anything, CON programs tended to increase costs."[24] Several factors doomed CON, starting with the politics of the HSAs. Providers made up nearly half of each HSA, and they tended to support each other's CON applications on a quid pro quo basis. Hence, proposals needed the support of only a few other HSA members to win approval. Other HSA members were inclined to support proposals as well, realizing that most proposals provided a tangible benefit to the local Health Services Area, but most of the cost was shared nationwide through Medicare and Medicaid.

There were other problems with CON. Providers often submitted multiple CON applications to make sure that at least one was approved. This proved to be an administrative burden for both providers and regulators, and one that went far to defeat the purpose of CON. Most significantly, CON did not apply to physicians or outpatient facilities. This exemption was a major catalyst for the growth of outpatient diagnostic and surgical services, as physicians eagerly filled the void in those instances when HSAs denied hospital requests for CON.

By the mid-1980s, many policy makers questioned the value of facilities planning. Not only did the evidence suggest that planning did not matter. The underlying rationale for the planning regulations—market failure—seemed less of a concern. HCFA's PPS and managed care were directly addressing inefficiencies in the traditional health economy. At the same time, Ronald Reagan had put an end to the era of big government. In 1986, the federal government repealed PL 93-641. Since then, twelve states have repealed all or part of their local CON laws, while others took the teeth out of theirs. A 1998 study by Christopher Conover and Frank Sloan finds no evidence of any increase in facilities acquisition or in total health care spending following these repeals.[25] While most states continue to require CON for selected services, especially long-term care, facilities planning is largely dead.

Manpower Planning Revisited

Unlike facilities planning, manpower planning has not falle_
out of fashion. In his national health insurance plan, Bill Clinton proposeu
to correct a perceived imbalance in the numbers of generalist and specialist physicians in the United States. (The ratio of generalists to specialists
in the United States is 1 to 2; in most other nations it is closer to 2 to 1.)
Many economists have argued that the prevalence of specialists in the
United States reflects patient demand for high-quality physician services.
Planners counter that patient demand is often inappropriate, due to demand inducement and moral hazard. In their view, the demand for specialists unnecessarily drives up already high medical care costs.

Under the Clinton plan, a government agency would have allocated residency training spots to hospitals, with the goal of restricting specialty training and boosting generalist training. As with previous planning efforts,
however, market forces are already at work toward the same ends. As a
result of managed care, the earnings of generalists are rising relative to
those of specialists.[26] This, in turn, has encouraged more medical school
graduates to pursue residency training in primary care. (Managed care is
apparently also behind the 17 percent decline in medical school applications between 1996 and 1999.[27]) Ironically, even as the government seeks
to reduce the number of specialists, it provides a $6 billion annual subsidy
to specialists training through the Medicare program. This works out to
roughly $100,000 per resident annually and surely contributes to the rela-
tively high number of specialists in the United States. It is somewhat numb-
ing to think that we would need a government program to correct the
"problem" of specialist oversupply that itself is the result of another government program. In such ways, one regulatory program begets another.

Efforts to Improve Quality

Through rate review and CON, planners hoped to reduce prices and quan-
tities. Through Professional Standards Review Organizations, established
in 1972, they hoped to boost quality. PSROs were local organizations of
physicians charged with monitoring the necessity, appropriateness, and
quality of care provided to hospitalized Medicare and Medicaid patients.[28]
PSROs established standards of care for a wide range of diseases and
could direct HCFA to withhold payment from physicians whose treatment
decisions did not measure up to these standards.

PSROs, which represented the first major effort by the government to
directly monitor quality, proved to be ineffective. It took more than five

years for most PSROs to form, and even longer for them to establish standards. PSROs were reluctant to penalize physicians who were statistical "outliers" and rarely took action beyond withholding payments on a case-by-case basis. PSROs were replaced in 1983 by Professional Review Organizations, which are private organizations employed by HCFA to assure the necessity and appropriateness of Medicare services and to review medical records for evidence of excessive upcoding, dumping, and unbundling of services. Many PROs have been instrumental in developing methods for utilization review (UR) that have been copied by private insurers. I will discuss UR at length in the next chapter.

UNINTENDED CONSEQUENCES: THE RISE OF INVESTOR-OWNED SYSTEMS

Although pricing and planning regulation did little to stem the growth of health care costs, they catalyzed another important change in the health economy—the growth of for-profit hospital chains. For-profit hospitals were actually quite prevalent in the first half of the century. In 1928, the first year for which such data are available, there were about nineteen hundred for-profit community hospitals, versus about eight hundred today.[29] The typical for-profit hospital was owned by a doctor (or a small group of doctors), was situated in a small town, and had fewer than one hundred beds.

After World War II, nonprofit hospitals proliferated. Thanks to major scientific advances in anesthetics and antibiotics, the demand for hospital care grew rapidly. Many communities took over their local for-profit hospitals, converted them to nonprofit status, and infused much-needed cash into aging facilities. The 1946 Hill-Burton Act pumped more money into nonprofits, providing $3.7 billion for the construction and improvement of nonprofit hospitals between 1947 and 1971. Local and state matching funds added another $9.1 billion.

By the 1970s, the small, rural, for-profit hospitals were in trouble. They could not access the capital available to nonprofits; they lacked the accounting skills necessary to exploit the loopholes of cost-based reimbursement; and they were unable to navigate the red tape of planning laws. These for-profits turned to national, investor-owned systems for help.

Essentially nonexistent prior to 1970, the investor-owned systems, including Hospital Corporation of America (the precursor to Columbia/HCA), Humana, National Medical Enterprises (NME), and American Medical International (AMI), acquired over 100 hospitals by 1975. By 1980, the systems owned 273 hospitals; by 1985, they owned nearly 500 hospitals and managed, under contract, 200 more. The systems brought much-needed efficiencies to the hospitals that they controlled. They exploited their access to capital markets to upgrade facilities; standardized systems for accounting, billing, purchasing, and hiring, and for coping with regulatory requirements; used their size to obtain better prices for medical supplies; took advantage of market power and knowledge of consumer demand by raising prices whenever possible; and offered promotion opportunities for skilled managers. These efficiencies enabled the systems to achieve a healthy 12 percent pretax return on equity through the 1970s and 1980s.

It is difficult to overstate the hostility with which the mainstream health care community reacted to the success of the investor-owned systems. When I was a health services management student in the late 1970s, several of my professors at Cornell complained that the health care marketplace would quickly be dominated by a handful of for-profit systems. My professors were not alone in fearing what Paul Starr called "the coming of the corporation." Paul Ellwood gloomily predicted that, by 1990, ten to twenty chains would control the health care of 60 percent of Americans.[30] Senator Howard Metzenbaum snapped at a for-profit hospital executive, "You and your organizations have taken the side of private greed."[31] In a famous article in the *New England Journal of Medicine* in 1980, journal editor Arnold Relman captured the feelings of many physicians, stating that the commercialism of medicine was creating a "medical-industrial complex."[32]

These critics were afraid that hospital managers would place the interests of investors above those of patients. At a minimum, this would mean that uninsured patients might not find a private hospital willing to treat them. But for-profit medicine was deemed a threat to all patients. As Mechanic has argued, it boils down to whether patients can trust in the compassion of for-profits: "Although there are many responsible (for-profit) companies, others seek quick profits and engage in dishonest practices."[33] To many Americans, for-profit medicine represented the opposite extreme of Marcus Welby medicine, with greed overtaking compassion as the driving force in the health economy.

These fears proved to be unwarranted. The investor-owned hospitals' share of the overall hospital marketplace started falling in the mid-1980s and bottomed out in the early 1990s. HCA, which owned over 200 hospitals in 1985, had only 80 by 1992. AMI had shrunk from 90 to 35; Humana, which had owned over 80 hospitals in the mid-1980s, totally divested its hospital ownership. There was a brief resurgence of national for-profit systems in the mid-1990s, when Richard Scott's small Columbia Healthcare System acquired much larger chains to eventually create Columbia/HCA. There was a sense of déjà vu as some analysts in the early 1990s forecast that Columbia/HCA and other chains would soon dominate the health economy. In the wake of HCFA investigations into its Medicare billing practices, and difficulties competing in urban markets, Columbia began to sell off its urban hospitals in 1998. Today, the largest for-profit chain is the Quorum Health Group, which owns nearly 300 hospitals. Tenet, the result of a merger between NME and AMI, is the only other chain that owns over 100 hospitals.

Several factors contributed to the lackluster performance of for-profit systems. Systems that wanted to expand had to find willing sellers. Once the systems had bought out the doctor-owned for-profits, they had to turn to the nonprofits. But most nonprofits were doing rather well financially and had no reason to sell. To cope with new regulations, the larger nonprofits had obtained managerial expertise on their own. An important step was the hiring of professional managers, many of whom have degrees from top graduate business schools. (For example, the CEOs of Chicago's top hospitals and systems, including Northwestern Memorial Hospital, the University of Chicago Hospital, Evanston Hospital, and the Advocate Health Care system, all have MBAs.) Nonprofits also benefited from the proliferation of consulting firms specializing in health care. These firms helped nonprofits improve administrative functions such as billing and personnel management. To reap the benefits of economies of scale, nonprofits partnered to form national alliances. The three largest alliances merged in 1996; the resulting Premier Health Alliance has over 1,700 hospitals. Through Premier and other alliances, nonprofits can match the efficiencies of for-profit systems in areas such as purchasing, accounting, marketing, planning, and staffing. Several research studies have confirmed that nonprofit hospitals are just as efficient as for-profits.[34] With nothing to gain by way of efficiencies, and much to lose in terms of fulfilling their missions, most nonprofits rejected the overtures of the systems.

For-Profit Branding Strategies

Unable to grow by acquiring nonprofits, investor-owned systems turned to other growth strategies. One of the most highly publicized was an effort in the 1980s by Humana to establish a brand-name identity. Humana was unique among the for-profit systems in that all of its hospitals shared the same corporate name, for example, Humana Hospital–Brazos Valley (Texas) and Humana Hospital–Springhill (Louisiana). At best, the other for-profit systems, such as AMI and HCA, tacked their corporate logo onto the established name of the hospitals they owned; hence, AMI Mission Bay Hospital in San Diego and HCA Valley Regional Medical Center in Brownsville, Texas. Humana pushed the branding concept further by opening a national chain of over 150 Humana MedFirst clinics. Through this brand-name extension, Humana hoped to attract primary care patients who would eventually be referred to their specialists and fill their hospital beds. By the mid-1980s, Humana was spending $30 million annually to promote its brand on billboards, radio, and television.

Humana's branding efforts failed. Claiming that its cookie-cutter approach to medicine resembled the retailing of fast food, critics referred derisively to Humana's MedFirst offices as "docs in the box." Local physicians viewed the clinics as direct competitors for primary care business, discouraged patients from visiting the clinics, and refused to refer patients to Humana hospitals. To make matters worse, Humana plowed administrative personnel into the clinics, thus forgoing opportunities to enjoy scale economies. When the clinics struggled, Humana hospitals failed to gain share against their "unbranded" competitors. Humana had made a fatal mistake: it tried to establish a national brand for a product for which national branding would not work.

In general, national brands tend to fall into three categories. Some, such as Intel and Sony, connote quality across their product lines. No one believed that Humana offered superior quality; if anything, Humana was fighting a perception of inferior quality. Other brands, such as Budweiser and Coke, have images and emotions—sex, youth, wealth—attached to their products. But most patients do not want to feel sexy, youthful, or wealthy in conjunction with their hospital stay; they just want to get better. Other national brands, such as Home Depot and McDonalds, are chain stores. Branding helps them in two ways. First, they enjoy marketing economies through national advertising. Second, consumers value their uniform appearance, quality, and selection and readily shop at any store in the chain. Humana could have placed national ads, but why would it want to? With fewer than one hundred hospitals, it was absent from most major markets, including New York, Philadelphia, Detroit, and San Francisco. At the same time, it is doubtful that consumers wanted uniformity in the provision of health care. In fact, Humana MedFirst failed partly because of its uniformity and the associated negative connotations.

THE GOVERNMENT AS AGENT

Through regulations to expand access and reduce costs, federal and state governments have made their mark on the patient's shopping problem. Initially, Medicare and Medicaid were intended to be "hands-off" insurance programs. They were modeled after traditional indemnity plans in which recipients could freely choose their providers, and providers could have unfettered control over medical decision making. But in the name of cost containment and quality control, Medicare and Medicaid have used many of the same strategies adopted by managed care. Sometimes, Medicare and Medicaid are the first to introduce these strategies. Through rate setting, Medicare provides financial incentives for providers to limit inpatient utilization. Through PRSOs and PROs, Medicare reviews and occasionally rejects treatment plans. And both Medicare and Medicaid are increasingly shifting enrollees into MCOs.

Another way that regulation affects patient shopping is by limiting the choice of provider. For example, one of the goals of PL 93-641 was to limit the availability of sophisticated medical technologies to a handful of regional centers that might better exploit scale economies. To accomplish this, HSAs tried to concentrate services in a select few hospitals. This restriction on access is similar to current MCO policies that direct patients to low-cost "preferred providers." Regulation limits access to providers in other ways. Recent federal manpower planning proposals would have reduced the number of available specialists and designated where they could receive their training. State cutbacks in Medicaid payments to providers have caused many providers to refuse to treat Medicaid patients. Comparable reductions in Medicare payments, which Congress has considered as a way to keep Medicare spending in check, would presumably lead to the same access problems.

Recently, some states have enacted laws intended to counter perceived access restrictions imposed by managed care. As of 1999, sixteen states required a minimum stay for mastectomy patients, and forty-two states had rules governing "drive-through deliveries." For now, these restrictions have little practical importance. For example, when the Illinois legislature debated its ban on outpatient mastectomies, it was observed that all mastectomies in the state were performed as inpatient procedures. But as technology evolves, practices that are considered dangerous today may become both feasible and appropriate. Consider that at one time it was inconceivable that patients could have their appendixes removed or their hernias repaired without spending several days in the hospital. These are now the bread and butter of outpatient surgery. Yet imagine the extra cost and inconvenience to patients today if, two decades ago, well-intentioned legislators had passed laws banning "drive-through" appendectomies and hernia surgery. There is every reason to believe that as medical science continues to advance, procedures that are currently done on an inpatient basis, such as mastectomies, will be safely, conveniently, and efficiently performed on an outpatient basis—unless, of course, regulatory practice restrictions stand in the way.

NATIONAL HEALTH INSURANCE AND THE SHOPPING PROBLEM

Since the inception of Medicare and Medicaid, federal and state governments have repeatedly tried to eliminate inefficiencies in the traditional health economy. Some interventions, such as the PPS, appear to have enjoyed some success. (At the very least, PPS reduced inpatient costs.) Some, such as manpower planning, may have done more harm than good. Others, such as facilities planning, were mainly a waste of time and effort.

It is easy to criticize the mixed track record of government intervention and call for the government to keep out of the health economy. But the government intervened in the health economy for much the same reasons that managed care emerged—the widespread perception that the traditional health economy was inefficient. Perhaps planning failed to contain costs because it was poorly implemented. Or maybe planners left too many resource allocation decisions in the hands of providers and patients. Maybe it takes a fully regulated health economy, such as in Canada, to rein in costs. After all, Canadians spend one-third less on their health care than do Americans, yet most Canadians appear to be very satisfied with their single-payer system.

This begs a question: What is the difference between free-market efforts to eliminate inefficiency, such as managed care, and government efforts, such as a single-payer system? Every year, I pose this question to my students. To help them answer it, I play a simple game, in which I describe a health care "system" with the following features:

- The payer dictates the prices it will pay to physicians and other providers.
- The payer controls capital growth by reviewing all requests for new equipment and facilities.
- The payer refuses to pay for certain costly services of questionable medical value.

I ask students to name the system. Several students identify this as the Canadian single-payer system, or perhaps the British National Health Service. After additional thought, however, others suggest the system I have in mind is the Kaiser Foundation Health Plan. The point of this game is that they are all correct. There are, in fact, many similarities between the Canadian and British systems and my hypothetical system. But Kaiser's approach to solving problems in the traditional health economy is similar to that taken by many national systems. (Kaiser's costs also approach those in national systems.)

So what is the difference between a market-based approach and a regulatory approach to improving the health economy? One difference is that it is easier to extend health insurance coverage to the entire population using a regulatory approach. But there have been many proposals for expanding insurance coverage through the marketplace, including Enthoven's Consumer Choice Health Plan and Clinton's National Health Security Act. My simple game highlights a more subtle but potentially more far-reaching difference. Each insurance plan in a market-based system can offer its own distinct solution to the shopping problem. Consumers who are not satisfied with, say, the Kaiser solution can shop around for a plan that tries a different solution. Consumer choice therefore has the potential to create powerful incentives for MCOs to find innovative ways to eliminate waste and improve quality. Under a single-payer system, consumers do not have a choice of solutions. Moreover, bureaucrats may have less incentive to find the best solutions because they have little to gain from innovative ideas. At the same time, powerful interest groups may exert undue influence on how the system is organized.

Lest one think that the choice between a market-based system and a single-payer system clearly favors the former, remember that the powerful incentives created by consumer choice are not always in evidence in health care markets—important innovations such as prospective payment and utilization review were initiated by the government. Moreover, consumer choice comes at a cost. Choice means competition. In competing to sign up enrollees, insurers advertise and deploy large sales forces. They also engage in "medical underwriting," in which they attempt to forecast the medical needs of specific enrollees so as to better set premiums. One need only compare the administrative costs of Medicare (on the order of 3 to 4 percent of program costs)[35] with those of MCOs (on the order of 10 to 15 percent of costs or higher) to get a handle on the cost of marketing and underwriting.[36] Some believe that medical underwriting is unfair as well as costly because as it drives up insurance premiums for very sick individuals and leaves some with no insurance whatsoever. A single-payer system avoids these problems. There is one additional drawback to the market-based approach: many consumers do not choose their own plan. Instead, their employer does. As I will discuss later, employers do not necessarily choose the plan that best serves the needs of their employees.

For the foreseeable future, the American public appears willing to accept the shortcomings of market-based health care. Managed care seems to have accomplished what regulation could not—stem the rising cost of medical care. But has the market really motivated managed care plans to solve the problems of the health economy? Do managed care plans really lower costs? Or do they merely sign up low-cost enrollees? Do they really manage care? Or have they found shortcuts that allow them to cut costs at the expense of quality? To answer these questions, we must explore the recent history of managed care.

CHAPTER 4

Managed Care Takes Over

BY THE EARLY 1980s, the U.S. health economy was in turmoil. The government planning efforts of the 1970s had failed to curtail cost inflation, and national health expenditures continued to show double-digit annual increases. By 1982, health expenditures had risen to more than 10 percent of the GDP and were forecast to rise steadily. By 1990, health care accounted for 12.6 percent of the GDP, and some analysts predicted that figure would exceed 20 percent by the year 2000. (The current figure is under 14 percent.)

Although much of the burden of rising costs fell squarely on the firms that purchased private health insurance, most were doing little about it. Employers reasoned that when it came to health care costs, all firms were in the same boat. Moreover, the cost of health care seemed to be largely beyond their control. It made sense for businesses to let the federal government take a stab at cost containment. But double-digit annual cost increases eventually took their toll on employers. As early as the mid-1970s, some employers complained that rising health care costs put them at a competitive disadvantage when compared with firms in other countries—health care costs in Canada, Europe, and Japan were 25 to 50 percent less than in the United States and were paid for by the government. Despairing about the competitiveness of the U.S. auto industry in 1976, a top official at General Motors observed that Blue Cross and Blue Shield had become a larger supplier to GM than U.S. Steel.[1] As costs continued to mount in the 1980s, many firms found they were spending close to 10 percent of their labor costs on health insurance. Even firms insulated from foreign competition began to fret. By 1989, 60 percent of corporate executives responding to a Robert Wood Johnson Foundation survey labeled health care costs a "major concern," and 35 percent called them a "top concern."[2] The failure of government cost containment efforts forced businesses to seek their own solution.

The only solution that the private sector had to offer was managed care. Yet outside of a few geographic pockets (mainly the West Coast and Minnesota), managed care was not even on the radar screen of most business executives, and for good reason. HMO enrollments in the mid-1970s just surpassed 5 million, and that included 2 million in the California Kaiser plans. For most of the nation, managed care was dismissed as a "West Coast thing." That would soon change.

CHAMPIONS OF THE HMO MOVEMENT

During the 1970s, a small but influential group of mainly West Coast business leaders and academics, led by Paul Ellwood, Alain Enthoven, and Harold Luft, began spreading the word about HMOs. Ellwood, trained as a primary care physician, had been a backer of HMOs since the 1960s and was influential in shaping President Nixon's plan for national health insurance, a plan that would have placed most Americans in an HMO. His consulting firm, Interstudy, was the first to gather widespread data about HMOs. Enthoven introduced cost-benefit analysis to President Kennedy's Department of Defense, and as a trustee of Georgetown University, he helped form the University Hospital's first HMO. His interest in HMOs grew when, while attending a 1971 national health care conference in Aspen, Colorado, he met Paul Ellwood on the way to the ski slopes. In 1973, he joined the faculty at Stanford University's Graduate School of Business, where he began a consulting relationship with Kaiser-Permanente. By the end of the 1970s, Enthoven had published articles in prominent journals about flat-of-the-curve medicine and developed the Consumer-Choice Health Plan (CCHP), a national health insurance plan based on market principles. CCHP received considerable support in Congress but was ultimately rejected by President Reagan, perhaps because of the cost required to include the uninsured in the plan. During this time, Enthoven conducted research with Luft, an economist at the University of California, San Francisco. Luft and Enthoven's research highlighted some of the inefficiencies in the health economy. In 1978, Luft independently published his pathbreaking research about HMOs.[3]

To promote HMOs as an alternative to indemnity insurance, Enthoven and Paul Ellwood met with local business groups, including many regional Business Groups on Health, and presented their ideas to receptive business leaders at conferences and in boardrooms. Ellwood invited leaders from the private sector to his vacation condo in Jackson Hole to talk about HMOs, while Enthoven used his position as a chaired business school professor to lend credibility to the HMO movement.

In 1992, Ellwood invited dozens of academics and business leaders to his Wyoming home for a series of meetings to discuss national health insurance. (By then, Ellwood had built a larger home to accommodate his guests.) The Jackson Hole Group ultimately played a major role in the national health insurance debate of the early to mid-1990s. Led by Enthoven, the group developed a national health insurance plan based on principles of "managed competition," and Bush administration officials were frequent guests at group meetings.[4]

In their efforts to promote the growth of HMOs, Enthoven and Ellwood were aided by an unlikely ally—Blue Cross. The Blues were typically the leading indemnity insurers in their markets. Originally organized by local providers, the Blues had been steadfastly opposed to managed care, but in a 1967 speech to Blue Cross Association members, the association's recently appointed president, Walter McNerny, surprised his audience by supporting research and discussions about prepaid group practices. Afterward, he stated, "If the conference accomplished anything, it was to make group practice a legitimate subject for conversation."[5]

McNerny's speech created a small division between insurers and providers, one that would ultimately turn into a chasm. While the American Medical Association reiterated its objections to prepaid group practice and the Public Health Service turned down a Blue Cross Association proposal to fund research into group practice, McNerny prodded local plans to establish HMOs. By 1973, there were six operational Blue Cross HMOs, and by 1980 the Blue Cross HMOs in California, Ohio, Illinois, and elsewhere were among the largest in the nation. These plans lent legitimacy to the HMO concept and gave employers the option of contracting with a nonprofit HMO whose brand name was acceptable to employees. Thanks in no small part to the national efforts of Ellwood, Enthoven, Luft, McNerny, and countless other "evangelists" in local markets, business leaders gradually came to accept HMOs. HMO enrollments increased steadily throughout the 1980s, from 9.1 million in 1980 to 33.6 million in 1990. Fueled by rising demand, new HMOs popped up everywhere. There were fewer than 100 HMOs in 1980; less than a decade later, there were more than 600. Today, over 60 million Americans are enrolled in over 500 HMOs, and more than 80 percent of working Americans are enrolled in some kind of managed care plan. The "West Coast thing" has spread across the nation.

Regional Differences in HMO Growth

HMO growth through the 1980s was uneven. Already firmly established on the West Coast, by the end of the decade HMOs had a strong presence in upstate New York, New England, and the upper Midwest. Many factors contributed to the uneven growth. HMOs thrived in markets where physicians were already organized into groups and where there was a history of cooperation among providers, as in Seattle and Rochester, New York. They also did better in markets with excess hospital capacity, which enabled HMOs to strike better deals for hospital services.

In a few communities, employers have been especially aggressive in promoting the growth of managed care. Nowhere have employers been more involved in shaping their health care marketplace than in the Twin Cities of Minneapolis–St. Paul. Employers in the Twin Cities were among the first outside of the West Coast to embrace HMOs. In the 1970s, HMO enrollment in the Twin Cities grew at an annual rate in excess of 20 percent. By the end of the 1980s, over half of the local population belonged to HMOs. In 1988, a coalition of twenty-four of the largest Twin Cities employers went beyond merely offering their employees a choice of HMOs and formed the Business Health Care Action Group (BHCAG). Originally formed to lobby for health care reform, by 1991 the BHCAG was purchasing managed care plans on behalf of nearly twenty-five local businesses. In 1997, BHCAG found that mergers among HMOs and PPOs had reduced its managed care options to just three competitors. BHCAG bypassed the established MCOs and created its own health plan by directly contracting with local health systems and physician networks. Today, BHCAG publishes a guide that enables employees to evaluate each local physician group on a variety of measures of quality as well as price. BHCAG has also developed and implemented treatment guidelines aimed at improving quality.

BHCAG had initial success with direct contracting, securing 10 percent reductions in insurance costs in the first year. But it turned out that providers had set unrealistically low prices and suffered substantial losses on the BHCAG contract. The three largest health systems in the Twin Cities raised prices by an average of 20 percent in 1998, followed by a more modest increase in 1999. Still, it appears that the rate of growth of BHCAG costs lags behind that for similar firms in Minnesota purchasing traditional MCO plans. It is too soon to be certain whether BHCAG has accomplished anything more than concentrate purchasing power and arouse the anxiety of Twin Cities providers. But the BHCAG model, in which a group of local employers uses economic and clinical data to guide plan and provider selection, is likely to be replicated elsewhere.

FORMS OF MANAGED CARE

The HMOs that emerged during the 1980s did not always resemble the prepaid group practices embodied by Kaiser and the Group Health Cooperative of Puget Sound. To distinguish among the various types of HMOs, Paul Elwood has grouped them into four categories based on how the physicians are organized: staff model, group model, independent practice association (IPA), and network model. Staff model HMOs are insurance companies that employ their physicians. Because they receive a salary, physicians in these HMOs have no direct financial incentive to induce demand or cater to patient moral hazard. Group model HMOs are insurance companies that contract with large physician groups to provide professional and, occasionally, ancillary services. The most successful early HMOs, including Kaiser and the Group Health Cooperative, were typically either a staff or a group model. Physicians in staff and group models often work exclusively for the HMO. Both staff and group model HMOs may restrict where physicians can hospitalize their patients.

Kaiser-Permanente plans have features common to both group and staff model HMOs. Each regional plan contracts with the local Permanente medical group to provide all physician services at Kaiser-owned facilities. The group agrees to treat only Kaiser patients. The plan pays the group a fixed fee per enrollee, and the group, in turn, pays a salary to each member. After a few years with the group, each member may become a partner and receive a share of group profits. There are some differences between Kaiser-Permanente and other group models. Most other physician groups contract with more than one HMO. Physicians in other groups do not always receive a fixed salary; some groups pay their members on a fee-for-service basis. Some groups use complex bonus schemes based on patient satisfaction, reenrollment, and other measures of performance.

In 1980, staff and group model HMOs accounted for 60 percent of all HMOs and had over 80 percent of HMO enrollees. Physicians committed to the idea of prepayment were usually the ones to start staff and group model HMOs. As employers sought out HMOs, most physicians remained stubbornly resistant to prepayment, and few new staff and group models emerged during the 1980s. The surging demand for HMOs would have to be met by other forms.

IPAs and network model HMOs have built on the existing provider infrastructure. They are often little more than a nexus of contracts between insurers and providers, without much brick and mortar to show for them. Many IPAs were formed by groups of physicians who wanted to retain their current practice style and their independence. Their IPAs acted as insurance companies, collecting fixed fees per enrollee and making payments to IPA members. Curiously, most of the early IPAs paid their members on a fee-for-service basis, thus failing to reverse the incentives of traditional indemnity insurance. Not surprisingly, many of the early IPAs had very high costs and went out of business. Network model HMOs were formed by regional and national insurers eager to meet the demand for HMOs by their largest employer/customers. These insurers (which included the Blues, Aetna, and Prudential) contracted with individual physicians and physician groups in private practice. They permitted physicians to contract with several HMOs and to maintain their non-HMO practice. Many network insurers paid physicians on a fee-for-service basis, but they usually managed to secure discounts off of the physicians' usual fees.

IPAs, networks, and other "mixed models" (models that combine features of IPAs and networks) enjoyed the greatest growth among HMOs. In 1980, there were ninety-seven IPA, network, and mixed plans with 1.7

million enrollees; there are now over four hundred of these plans, with nearly 50 million enrollees. Patients prefer them over staff and group model HMOs because they cause the least disruption to the traditional health economy; physicians like them for the same reason. Regional and national employers especially like the plans offered by regional and national insurers because these plans offer the convenience of one-stop shopping. All these factors help explain why HMOs organized by regional and national insurers, many of which are for-profit, have grown so rapidly.

In addition to securing physician services, HMOs must arrange for hospital and other medical services. Some staff and group model HMOs, including the GHC and Kaiser, own their own hospitals. Most other HMOs contract with a subset of hospitals in their local markets and direct their physicians to admit patients to them. By the 1970s, some non-HMO insurers discovered that they could reduce their costs by pursuing the same strategy of contracting with selected hospitals. These were among the first preferred provider organizations (PPOs).

Preferred Provider Organizations

According to economist Ted Frech, the earliest PPO may have been a Los Angeles firm, Dual-Plus, which "contracted with a panel of physicians on behalf of some insurance firms in 1970."[6] In 1978, AdMar, a third-party administrator (TPA) for employers offering their own health plans, began selectively contracting with Los Angeles area hospitals. In what became a model for PPOs, AdMar secured discounts from the contracting hospitals. To encourage hospitals to give discounts, AdMar required employees to make a copayment when visiting noncontracting hospitals; this motivated employees to visit the "preferred" hospitals. Frech reports that the name "PPO" was first used by Linda Ellwein, a member of Interstudy, Paul Ellwood's think tank.

Despite early successes, PPOs faced a serious regulatory obstacle. Every state had laws requiring that insurers provide the same contractual terms to all providers. Among other things, this meant that insurers could not refuse to reimburse for services from some providers while reimbursing for the same services provided by others. This would render PPOs impotent; if they could not exclude some providers from their contracts, they could not boost volumes for other providers, and thus no provider would have an incentive to lower its price or adopt a less costly practice style to become a "preferred provider." By the mid-1980s, however, states were removing this regulatory barrier. Beginning with California in 1982, most states rewrote their insurance laws to permit selective contracting by insurers. The California legislation explicitly stated that the purpose of the rewritten law was to promote competition and lower prices. It worked. By 1984, the low prices secured by Blue Cross's Prudent Buyer PPO enabled it to sign up five hundred thousand members, and several other PPOs had formed within the state.

Many employers did not wait for the laws to change before offering PPOs to their employees. Thanks to a relatively obscure provision in the 1974 federal Employee Retiree Income and Security Act (ERISA), self-funded employer-sponsored health insurance plans were exempt from state insurance regulation, including mandated benefit design and bans on selective contracting.[7] Self-insured firms rely on TPAs like AdMar to assist with all aspects of self-insurance, including selective contracting. By the early 1980s, many firms were self-insuring to avoid state regulations, and selective contracting was an attractive option to those self-insured firms seeking to further reduce insurance costs. Today, over 70 percent of firms with over five hundred employees offer a self-insured plan to their employees. Working with TPAs, most of these firms offer a PPO option.

Though once scorned as "halfhearted" HMOs—they impose only some of the access restrictions common among HMOs—PPOs have been very successful. They were nonexistent in 1980 and were barely on the radar screen in 1986. Today, however, estimates of PPO enrollments range from 50 million (Health Insurance Association of America estimate) to nearly 100 million (American Association of Health Plans estimate).[8] PPO enrollments continue to grow, and with so few Americans left in indemnity plans, this growth comes mainly at the expense of HMOs. The fact that PPOs are "halfhearted" HMOs may explain their success. All else being equal, Americans prefer PPOs to HMOs because they are less intrusive.

Despite their success in the market, there are many complaints about PPO (and HMO) restrictions on access. Patients often must pay considerably more to visit a provider recommended by their PCP who is not in the MCO network. But it is at least theoretically possible that MCOs identify better providers than does the typical PCP, and it surely helps to hold down costs when the MCO, rather than the PCP, selects the referral network. Even so, the American public has never accepted MCO access restrictions, and politicians have scored easy political points by proposing "any willing provider" (AWP) legislation and "patient bill of rights" (PBR) laws that would limit the ability of MCOs to restrict access. But without the ability to restrict access, MCOs lose their leverage with providers. When providers know that they must be included in the network no matter what their practice style or price, they have no reason to make any concessions to MCOs. This is why states had to rewrite their insurance laws in the first place. (Unfortunately, recent studies of the effects of AWP and PBR legislation on health care costs have ignored this potential impact on competition.[9]) Unable to force managed care principles onto providers,

MCOs would quickly resemble indemnity plans.[10] For better or for worse, we would see the end of MCOs as we know them. Maybe that is the purpose of the legislation.

Point-of-Service Plans

One of the attractions of PPOs is that they usually provide some insurance coverage even if the patient does not visit a preferred provider. In this way, they give patients more "freedom of choice" than do most HMOs. In the past few years, some HMOs have introduced similar freedom of choice through what are cryptically known as "point-of-service" (POS) plans. Patients in a POS who go outside of the network of contracting providers may be reimbursed for half or more of the cost of treatment. There are roughly 10 million enrollees in POS plans, although enrollments seem to be declining.

MCO STRATEGIES

Managed care has become a catchall phrase, describing any insurance plan that impinges on the traditional medical care system. There are hundreds of managed care offerings, and the choices confronting employers and employees can seem bewildering. Yet MCOs rely on just three strategies for success: selective contracting, innovative incentives, and utilization review. To understand these strategies is to understand managed care.

Selective Contracting

Imagine what it would be like if consumers purchased automobiles the same way that they purchased health care services prior to managed care. Consumers would be responsible for selecting the car they wanted to buy, but "automobile insurance" would cover 80 to 100 percent of the price. Obviously, car makers would rejoice. They would surely raise prices, probably by quite a lot. After all, given that insurance was footing nearly all the bill, how many customers would care about price?

Luxury and exotic car manufacturers would be especially thrilled. A manufacturer like Mercedes that once had difficulty convincing customers to pay $50,000 for a car might easily be able to raise prices to $60,000, $70,000, or higher. Customers interested in buying a Mercedes might not even bother to shop around for competing models at lower prices because they would only stand to gain a small percentage of any price differential. Mercedes would not only enjoy higher prices; it might even ease up on the cost reduction programs that enabled it to remain price-competitive with other luxury nameplates. It could always raise its prices to cover the costs of any inefficiencies.

This bizarre scenario pretty much sums up the nature of price competition in the traditional health economy. Patients (and their PCPs) were largely responsible for selecting providers. But with insurance footing most of the bill, patients had little incentive to shop around for the best price. This alone would encourage providers to increase prices and pay a little less attention to costs. But additional factors took even more of the edge off of price competition in the health economy. Even if patients had an economic incentive to shop around for the best price, they often would have often done so under the duress of illness. On top of that, they would have been baffled by the prospect of comparing prices across providers. Providers did not price out treatments; instead, they priced individual services, such as a lab test, an office visit, and a minute in the operating room. This made comparison shopping for the best price almost impossible.

Mark Shanley, William White, and I describe the resulting competition among providers in the traditional health economy as "patient-driven."[11] Because patients were neither motivated to shop nor capable of shopping on the basis of price, the prices that providers set under patient-driven competition tended to vastly exceed the marginal cost of care. (In a perfectly competitive market, price equals marginal cost.) To make matters worse, providers were not overly concerned about staying efficient because they could always raise prices to cover their costs.

Insured patients may not have cared about the price of medical care, but the payers who had to foot the bill surely did. In the 1950s and 1960s, the Blues, Medicare, and Medicaid introduced cost-based reimbursement to limit price gouging. In the 1970s and 1980s, Medicaid and Medicare introduced rate setting. During this time, HMOs discovered that there was another way to pay lower prices for medical care. Rather than rely on accountants or regulators, they relied on the market. HMOs knew that insured patients would not discipline high-priced hospitals and physicians, so they did it themselves. HMOs negotiated with local hospitals and doctors and selectively contracted with those offering the best prices. At the same time, they refused to reimburse patients who sought care from noncontracting providers. By the early 1980s, indemnity insurers and self-funded employer plans also instituted selective contracting in PPOs.

Unlike patients, payers are highly motivated to get the best price they can because they get to keep any discounts. (To remain competitive in insurance markets, they may have to pass the savings along to enrollees.)

Payers are also better able to comparison shop. Because they are shopping on behalf of thousands of patients, payers can afford to employ contracting specialists. Through careful review of claims data, these specialists can compare prices that different providers charge for the same treatment and identify the lowest priced providers. Payers can credibly inform providers that if they do not give discounts, they will not get patients. To make this stick, they steer patients away from noncontracting providers (so-called out-of-network providers) by paying a much smaller portion of the medical bill. Shanley, White, and I describe the resulting competition among providers as "payer-driven."

Under payer-driven competition, providers are willing to give substantial discounts. They do so for the most fundamental of business reasons: to build market share or to avoid losing share. Under patient-driven competition, providers who offer discounts would have little to show for it besides lower revenues because few insured patients select their provider on the basis of price. But under payer-driven competition, price moves market share. Concerned about filling empty beds, some hospitals have given discounts of 50 percent or more to their most price-sensitive managed care purchasers, physicians often agree to discounts of 30 percent or more, and some drug manufacturers have given discounts of 80 percent or more to aggressive pharmacy benefits management companies to keep their products on formularies (lists of approved drugs).

Discounts vary in accordance with traditional economic theories of competition. Monopolists can resist discounting because payers have no choice but to contract with them. But sellers facing many close competitors (such as urban community hospitals) must set lower prices, especially if there is excess capacity in the market and each seller is fearful of losing market share.[12] Conversely, MCOs with substantial market shares can secure large discounts because many providers can ill afford to lose so many patients. It comes as no surprise that recent health care antitrust battles have pitted large, powerful providers against large, powerful payers.

Selective contracting appears to be all about getting lower prices. This creates the dangerous possibility that MCOs will steer patients to low-cost providers regardless of quality. But MCOs could, in principal, steer patients to the highest quality providers or to those offering the best value. Chapter 7 explores the potential for competition to bring out the very best from health care providers.

Innovative Incentives

Let us revisit the example of "automobile purchase insurance." Backed by insurance that promised to pay almost the entire price of a new car, few consumers would settle for a stripped-down Hyundai when they could own a fully loaded Mercedes or Lexus for just a few thousand dollars more. Naturally, spending on automobiles would skyrocket, but insurers would quickly catch on and take steps to reduce costs. An insurer might pay dealers a fixed price per car, regardless of the quality and options. Dealers would no longer sell luxury nameplates but instead might push Kias, Hyundais, and Saturns. Customers might object, and if they did not want a Kia, they would find another insurer. Of course, an insurer who was willing to pay for better quality cars would have to charge a higher premium.

Once again, there is a direct correspondence between this fiction of car buyers' insurance and the reality of the health economy. To control skyrocketing medical costs, many HMOs sever the link between compensation and utilization. The first prepaid group practices paid their physicians a fixed salary. Today's staff model HMOs do the same. In the short run, salaried physicians stand to make the same amount of money whether they provide "Lexus" treatment or "Hyundai" treatment.[13] This may incline physicians toward "Hyundai-style" undertreatment. This is not necessarily true in the long run, however, because HMOs can adjust annual salaries up or down based on physician performance. If an HMO rewards physicians who best contain costs, physicians will still be inclined toward undertreatment. On the other hand, if the HMO rewards physicians whose patients reenroll at the end of the year or report high rates of satisfaction, then physicians would be more likely to attend to their patients' needs. The HMOs would have to raise premiums to cover any attendant costs, however.

Another strategy that insurers use to rein in medical costs is to pay physicians a capitated fee. To understand how capitation works, imagine a small group of PCPs contracting with an HMO. The contract states that the PCPs must provide all medically necessary primary care at a capitated rate of $10 per member per month. During the HMO's annual sign-up period, one thousand members select physicians in that medical group to be their PCPs. The HMO thus pays the group $10,000 per month. In exchange, the group provides all necessary primary care for the one thousand members who select it.

Through capitation, insurers "push risk" onto providers. In other words, the HMO no longer suffers financially if a disproportionate percentage of the one thousand members turn out to be sick and require a lot of primary care. Instead, the PCPs bear the cost, which makes them sensitive to costs and presumably encourages them to limit utilization. But there are potential pitfalls to the HMO that adopts this strategy. The primary care group certainly has a financial incentive to reduce the utilization of its *own* services, but it has no incentive to reduce the utilization of any other services. The group might simply refer all of its patients to specialists. This could drive costs higher.

The HMO might address this problem by paying the group a higher capitated fee but requiring it to pay the costs of its referrals. For example, the HMO could pay $40 per member per month (or $40,000 total) to cover the cost of primary care and specialty care. Now, PCPs might think twice before referring patients to specialists. But new pitfalls appear. The HMO still must determine how to compensate specialists. If it pays them fee-for-service, then specialists will continue to have incentives to overtreat, much to the chagrin of PCPs. The HMO could capitate specialists, but this might discourage them from treating the most severely ill enrollees. There is a more subtle problem with capitation. PCPs might ignore their chronically ill patients altogether. Medical utilization by these patients eats into the capitated payment. PCPs may hope that if these patients are ignored they will select a different provider during the subsequent sign-up period. There is clearly no best way to use incentives to balance concerns about cost and quality. There are always trade-offs.

Capitation imposes another trade-off on physicians. By enabling physicians to profit by reducing utilization, capitation necessarily places them at financial risk. A few very sick patients can make a deep cut into a capitated physician's income. Like most people, physicians usually do not like to bear financial risk, and they will balk at a contract if the risk is extreme. This is why physicians have been reluctant to accept "global capitation" that would cover all physician, hospital, and outpatient care. Global capitation effectively turns physicians into insurance companies. Whereas an insurance company can spread risk across tens of thousands of enrollees, a few very sick patients can spell financial doom to an individual physician or insurer with a few hundred capitated patients.

This is the law of large numbers at work. By covering many patients, insurers are fairly certain that they will end up with an average number of very sick patients. By the same token, large capitated groups bear relatively little risk. Smaller groups and individually capitated physicians bear larger risks. Capitated individual specialists would bear the highest risks; they see fewer patients, a fraction of whom will have extraordinary medical needs. Clearly, the increased use of capitation favors larger groups, which are better able to bear the risk. But capitation of groups is no panacea for solving incentive problems. Large groups must still push the "right" incentives onto their member physicians. Groups may offer physicians a modified capitation, salary, fee-for-service payment, share of profits, or some other form of compensation. Groups may use promotions and end-of-year bonuses to reward "desired" performance. Just as is the case for HMO payments to physicians, each compensation method carries with it its own potentially conflicting incentives for efficiency and quality. There is no magic bullet.

Evidence on Incentives

No one doubts that health care providers respond to economic incentives. If there is a lot of money at stake, and a patient's condition falls in a gray area in which there is little to choose among alternative treatments, even Marcus Welby might place money above medicine and select the most remunerative treatment. Several researchers have sought to measure just how much incentives affect medical decision making. This seems like an easy task—researchers could ask providers how they would respond to different payment rules. A recent study did just that, randomly assigning internists to receive one of five questionnaires about ordering of medical services.[14] The questionnaires differed only in the type of reimbursement and utilization review. Physicians whose questionnaires depicted full capitation generally indicated that they would order fewer services than did physicians whose questionnaires indicated fee-for-service reimbursement.

Of course, it is difficult to be certain whether physicians will actually behave as they indicate in surveys. It would be preferable, therefore, to observe actual physician decision making. Alan Hillman, Mark Pauly, and Joseph Kerstein do this in a 1989 article in the *New England Journal of Medicine* and find that HMOs with capitated or salaried physicians had roughly 10 percent lower rates of hospital use than did insurers that made fee-for-service payments to physicians.[15] This result echoes Harold Luft's earlier findings about the difference between hospitalization rates at prepaid group practices and standard indemnity insurance plans. Thanks to studies such as these, there is a general consensus that the patients of capitated and salaried providers receive less medical care than do the patients of fee-for-service providers. The tempting conclusion is that the observed differences are due to incentives. This conclusion is premature, however, because of potential selection bias.

Two forms of selection bias plague studies of incentives. First, enrollees self-select. Enrollees in health plans that rely heavily on capitation (e.g., HMOs) are usually healthier than enrollees in plans that rely on fee-for-service reimbursement (PPOs and indemnity plans). Such self-selection is also possible among enrollees in different types of HMOs. As a result, we should expect the patients of capitated and salaried physicians to receive less care, regardless of provider incentives. Second, providers self-select. Providers with less aggressive treatment styles are more willing to participate in capitated plans; providers with more aggressive styles prefer fee-for-service plans. Provider self-selection would generate data consistent with the findings of Hillman, Pauly, and Kerstein's data, even if incentives do not change behavior.

In one remarkable study that overcomes objections about selection bias, the researchers randomly assigned residents in a teaching hospital to receive either a fee-for-service payment or a salary.[16] They also randomly assigned patients to residents. They find that patients of fee-for-service residents had about 20 percent more physician visits, mainly for well care. Randomized, controlled studies of economic behavior are rare, and this study remains unique. There is no other evidence on the effects of incentives on utilization that is fully immune to concerns about selection bias.[17] The bottom line is that incentives almost surely do matter, but no one knows exactly how much.

Such ignorance creates problems and opportunities for payers. The problem is that payers cannot anticipate *ex ante* how any particular payment scheme will affect utilization. From the provider's perspective, the design of payment schemes can therefore seem somewhat less than scientific, as payers grope around to find out what works best. But this gives payers an opportunity to collect data on their particular schemes, do some fine-tuning, and develop a payment approach that optimally balances cost containment and quality of care.

Even if MCOs find just the right mix of incentives to eliminate moral hazard and demand inducement without causing undertreatment, this will not be enough to assure that providers deliver efficient, effective health care. Incentives alone cannot assure that providers make the right medical decisions. Inspired by research on medical practice variations, MCOs complement the use of incentives by directly intervening in medical decision making.

Medical Practice Variations and Utilization Review

Beginning about three decades ago, health services researchers began to identify startling variations in medical practice across seemingly similar communities.[18] The research showed that the probability that patients received certain kinds of surgery, such as appendectomies, depended on where they lived. In a famous example, a research team led by Dartmouth University's Jack Wennberg reports that rates of certain procedures such as coronary artery bypass graft (CABG) surgery are much higher in New Haven than in Boston, but rates for other procedures such as carotid endarterectomy (a procedure to clear clogged arteries supplying the brain) are much higher in Boston.[19] Variations have been found for a wide range of interventions, from prostatectomies to cesarean sections, as well as for other medical services such as diagnostic testing and drug therapy. The *Dartmouth Atlas of Health Care*, edited by Wennberg, provides an in-depth look at practice variations across every hospital service area in the

United States.[20] It reports large practice variations for CABG, back surgery, angiography, and percutaneous transluminal coronary angioplasty (PTCA). Variations have also been found throughout the world. The extent of variations appears to be about the same in the United States as in Canada and Europe (although mean intervention rates are generally higher in the United States).

The magnitude of variations can be startling. One recent study found that the percentage of heart attack patients receiving beta-blockers at discharge from the hospital varied by region from under 10 percent to over 90 percent.[21] Most studies measure the extent of practice variations using a statistic called the coefficient of variation (CoV), which equals the standard deviation of the intervention rate across communities divided by the mean intervention rate.[22] Thus, if the mean annual rate of CABG surgery among Medicare patients is 6 per 1,000, and the standard deviation across communities is 2 per 1,000, then the CoV is 0.33. (These values are in line with those reported in research studies.[23]) This implies that in about one out of every six communities the CABG surgery rate is below 4 per 1,000, and in another one out of every six communities the rate exceeds 8 per 1,000. As reported by Charles Phelps, the CABG CoV of 0.33 is actually less than the CoV for many other costly interventions. For example, the CoV for knee replacement surgery has been estimated at 0.47, and the CoV for hip reconstruction was estimated at 0.69.

Differences in medical needs, demographics, and insurance coverage do not come close to fully explaining the variations. Rather, variations mainly seem to mainly reflect differences in the practice styles of physicians in different locales, or what economist Phelps and public policy analyst Cathleen Mooney call "divergent schools of thought" about the use of medical intervention.[24] Physicians develop their practice styles over many years, beginning in medical school and residency training. Some prefer treating certain illnesses aggressively, whereas others prefer a wait-and-see approach. Physicians may then congregate with others who have similar practice styles or may adjust their practice styles to resemble those of their colleagues. In doing so, physicians avoid conflict and increase the extent to which they learn from one another.

Just as physicians have different practice styles across communities, they also have different styles within communities. A study led by Phelps reports substantial differences in practice styles among physicians in Rochester, New York.[25] As Phelps puts it, "there turned out to be a wide array of 'styles' within this single medical community."[26] Because physicians have different practice styles, a patient who visits two physicians, either within the same community or especially in different communities, stands a good chance of obtaining two different diagnoses and/or two different treatment recommendations. The 1999 *Dartmouth Atlas of Health*

Care finds, for example, that less than 30 percent of women between the ages of sixty-five and sixty-nine receive mammograms with the recommended frequency, and even fewer receive the recommended colon cancer screens. Clearly, some providers are diligent about making sure that their patients receive these services, while others are lax. It is not as if physicians lack the opportunity to discuss the need for screening with their patients. Virtually all women in this age-group see physicians at least once a year for a variety of other health care needs. Reacting to this study, Christine Cassel, chair of the Department of Geriatrics at New York's Mount Sinai Hospital, observed, "Doctors know they're supposed to provide these services, and they don't."[27]

If one makes the reasonable presumption that there is some rate (or range of rates) of intervention that is appropriate, then large CoVs imply that all is not well with the current state of medical practice. Many patients are not getting needed interventions, while many others are receiving unnecessary care. This puts patients at risk, while also driving up costs. The medical risks are obvious in the case of patients who do not receive necessary care. But those who unnecessarily receive treatment are also harmed; many of the interventions with large CoVs are quite difficult, and some (such as CABG) have a nontrivial mortality risk. Phelps puts the total cost to the United States of variation in the use of CABG surgery at nearly $1 billion annually. (This includes the cost of unnecessary utilization and the cost of reduced health and lost productivity.) If we extrapolate this cost to all other hospital services, the cost of variations would easily exceed $10 billion annually.

The medical community is slowly waking up to the fact that, for now, unfettered physician decision making is not always optimal decision making. Citing a study on variations in treatment of heart attacks, Dr. David Meyerson of Johns Hopkins University notes that "the study underscores the need to get information on the best treatments to every corner of the medical community to get the best outcomes for our patients."[28] Cassel agrees that physicians lack the necessary information to schedule the appropriate treatments, stating, "We need to make this a no-brainer." By getting physicians to abide by appropriate norms of care, it should be possible to simultaneously reduce costs and improve outcomes. This is the premise behind one of the most important and controversial tools of managed care, utilization review.

How Utilization Review Works

Utilization review (UR) encompasses a variety of practices, including preadmission screening, to determine if the patient should enter the hospital or receive treatment elsewhere, surgical second opinion programs, and ongoing review of high-cost cases such as AIDS and cancer care. Supporters claim that UR assures that all patients will receive the proper interventions in the most appropriate settings. Detractors (especially physicians) view it as a convenient excuse for MCOs to cut costs at the expense of quality. To date, there is little systematic evidence to suggest that either side is correct.

Utilization review is not new. For decades, hospitals have performed their own internal UR. Each hospital's peer review committee examines selected medical charts to assure that the medical staff has provided competent care. Until recently, peer review committees focused exclusively on quality and did not address issues such as whether comparable quality could have been provided at a lower cost.

Formal external UR began with the federally sponsored PSROs. Based on reviews of the available clinical literature as well as discussions among experts, PSROs identified "best practices" for the treatment of a variety of illnesses. By reviewing patient records, PSROs identified outlier providers whose patients received care that departed significantly from best practice. In theory, the utilization levels of outlier providers could be either above or below the norms. In practice, PSROs seemed to focus their attention on providers whose utilization was above them. The same is true for the descendants of PSROs, including the Medicare PROs and private sector UR service agencies. Upon implementation of the Medicare PPS in 1983, the Health Care Finance Administration charged PROs with assuring the appropriateness of care. To achieve this end, PROs established elaborate guidelines and protocols to enforce them. Private health insurers quickly adopted similar practices; in fact, many private sector UR service agencies are outgrowths of Medicare PROs.

Interqual is the world's largest UR firm, providing services to PROs and private sector UR agencies. Its UR methods are representative of those of most other agencies. Medical staff at Interqual develop best practice criteria. The firm then compares actual practice with best practice to validate the appropriateness of hospitalizations, approve treatment plans, and monitor ongoing treatment of costly, chronic illnesses such as AIDS. Here is how it works for validation of hospitalizations (validation of surgery and chronic care is similar). Through evaluation of outcomes research and discussion with experts, Interqual develops illness-specific screens. It uses one set of screens to determine if the severity of illness is sufficient to warrant hospitalization and a second set to determine if it is appropriate and necessary to deliver the proposed treatment in a hospital.

When a physician wants to admit a patient to a hospital, the hospital's admissions nurse contacts Interqual. The nurse reports clinical information (symptoms, radiology and lab test results) and a treatment plan (diagnostic testing, surgery, intravenous fluid needs, and so forth). A nurse at Interqual runs this information through the two sets of screens and determines if the admission is appropriate. The Interqual nurse may recommend that the patient receive the treatment as an outpatient or may even refuse to accept the treatment plan. The hospital nurse and the admitting physician can challenge Interqual's recommendation, perhaps by presenting additional clinical information. In some cases, the admitting physician may discuss the case with a supervising physician at Interqual.

Does UR Work?

In theory, Interqual and other UR service firms create value by utilizing information about cost and quality based on careful, expert evaluations of outcomes research. This is not easy work. *Index Medicus* indexes articles in over thirty-three hundred medical journals. In any recent year, these journals will have contained literally hundreds of research studies on diseases such as prostate cancer and AIDS. Additional information is available at conferences where physicians present their latest clinical findings. Clearly, no one individual could hope to evaluate all this clinical information. Interqual and other UR service firms can afford these time-consuming evaluations because they can spread the costs across tens of thousands of patients who have the diseases. Ideally, the UR service firms would make the same choices that patients and their physicians would make if they had access to and understanding of the same information, and if they balanced costs against medical benefits. UR service agencies usually approve the proposed treatment plans or recommend lower cost alternatives, but they sometimes recommend more costly interventions. The idealized goal is not to reduce utilization across the board so much as to ensure that patients receive the right care.

Providers dismiss the possibility that UR service agencies diligently examine clinical research to develop state-of-the-art treatment plans that serve patient interests. Instead, they accuse the agencies of using simplified treatment criteria that ignore patients' idiosyncratic needs. UR service agencies are, of course, unwilling to reveal how they form their validation criteria. This is their sole source of competitive advantage, and it is not practical from a business perspective to release this information. Providers see UR agencies cloaked in secrecy and conclude that UR is an unwanted intrusion into clinical decision making motivated purely by the desire to generate profits for shareholders. Physicians even report that they would willingly lie about their patients' conditions if that would convince a UR firm to approve the proposed intervention.[29]

The idea that physicians would have to lie to obtain needed services appears to be damaging evidence of poor HMO quality. But physician complaints are somewhat disingenuous, particularly when it comes to preventive services. After studying comprehensive Medicare utilization data, Dartmouth's Wennberg finds that "HMOs, although they are targets of criticism on some issues, almost always have better performance records on screening tests than the traditional fee-for-service Medicare system."[30] It is harder to dismiss physician complaints about other treatments such as surgery. HMOs do occasionally reject physician treatment recommendations. But the theory and evidence on moral hazard, demand inducement, and practice variations suggest that physicians sometimes recommend the wrong treatments. If so, then perhaps physicians feel compelled to lie about their patients' conditions because the clinical information does not support the proposed interventions. Or do they need to lie because HMOs care only about costs and ignore patients' idiosyncratic needs altogether? No one really knows where the balance has been struck.

Unfortunately, there have been few published studies of the effectiveness of UR, and those studies usually confine themselves to the effects of UR on inpatient costs. For example, in a 1989 study, Thomas Wickizer, John Wheeler, and Paul Feldstein find that UR reduces inpatient costs by 10 percent.[31] In a 1998 study of a large psychiatric UR program, Wickizer and Daniel Lessler find that UR service agencies almost always approved requests for inpatient admissions but often refused to approve the requested lengths of stay.[32] They also find that patients who had shortened inpatient stays were slightly more likely to require readmission. Some evidence suggests that reductions in inpatient use are accompanied by increases in outpatient use. If so, it is not obvious whether UR restrictions on inpatient use save money.

The bottom line is that there are no studies to date that provide a definitive answer about how UR affects costs, nor are there any studies of whether UR systematically affects quality. This may explain why, in late 1999, United Healthcare decided to eliminate UR from its MCOs. Given that the purported goal of UR is to improve the appropriateness of medical care, it is imperative that research examine appropriateness rather than focus on costs. Thus far, such research is lacking.

As it turns out, there is a less intrusive alternative to UR. Rather than use norms to intervene in clinical decision making, MCOs can present the norms to providers and also identify physicians who are outliers. This is the approach that United Healthcare will pursue. Physicians can police themselves; for example, "outlier" physicians can change their practice patterns. If self-policing fails to rectify problematic practice patterns, then United and other MCOs can refuse to contract with physicians whose practice styles do not conform.

This information-based approach to controlling utilization is common in regulated health care systems and was even utilized by PSROs during the 1970s. Although the approach is popular among providers, especially when they participate in establishing the norms, there is no systematic evidence that it is any more or less successful than UR in controlling cost or boosting quality. It may turn out that MCOs will use information about practice styles when creating their networks, again engendering a negative reaction from providers. Even so, it seems like a less highly charged way for MCOs to introduce norms into clinical decision making than the direct intervention required by UR.

WHAT HAS MANAGED CARE ACCOMPLISHED?

MCOs grew out of an effort to eliminate the inefficiencies driving up the costs of the traditional health economy. The most obvious yardstick on which to measure the success of MCOs, therefore, is cost. But the great advantage of the traditional health economy was that economics never stood in the way of quality. If MCOs do cut costs, the resulting savings must ultimately be compared with any offsetting reductions in quality. Not surprisingly, there is a large and growing body of research assessing the effects of MCOs on both cost and quality.

Effects of Managed Care on Costs

The best evidence that managed care contains costs is that U.S. health care spending as a percentage of GDP peaked at 13.7 percent in 1993 and since then has stayed there or even declined slightly.[33] Spending in the year 2000 will be approximately $300 billion below projections made by the Congressional Budget Office in 1993. Medicare and Medicaid costs have generally risen faster than GDP, so the slowdown in the rate of growth of health care costs is largely attributable to managed care in the private sector. Even though private health insurance premiums (which are not the same as costs and tend to be more volatile) have risen substantially faster than the rate of inflation in each of the last two years, health care cost inflation is nowhere near the levels that were common prior to the growth of managed care. This casual empiricism is supported by a good deal of systematic economic research.

In a 1994 study, Robert Miller and Harold Luft reprise Luft's 1980 paper "How Do HMOs Achieve Their Savings?" Reviewing over a dozen studies published since 1980, they find that, compared with indemnity insurance, HMOs had lower inpatient utilization, similar or slightly higher outpatient utilization, and slightly lower costs.[34] These findings are consistent across all forms of HMOs, not just staff and group models. Just as Luft had done fourteen years earlier, Miller and Luft point out that the results might reflect selection bias.

Several excellent studies have appeared since 1994. A few compare health care costs in states that have experienced substantial managed care growth with costs in states with relatively little managed care. Such comparisons are largely immune to selection bias (assuming that unhealthy consumers do not move from state to state merely to avoid managed care). The studies unanimously find that managed care has contained the growth of health care costs. For example, David Cutler and Louise Sheiner examine changes in total health care spending in each state during the period 1988–93.[35] During this time, some states experienced rapid growth in managed care, whereas others did not. Cutler and Sheiner find that a 25 percentage point increase in managed care penetration (e.g., from 35 percent of the population to 60 percent) is associated with a 1 percent lower annual rate of growth of total health care spending. Other studies find that managed care leads to reductions in inpatient utilization, an increase in the number of primary care physicians, and fewer specialists. Studies confirm the bottom-line result of greatest interest, namely, managed care reduces health care costs.

MCOs may use any of three strategies for cost containment: selective contracting, innovative incentives, and UR. Which of these is most effective? The evidence clearly shows that selective contracting leads to lower prices, the evidence on incentives is weaker, and the evidence on UR is virtually nonexistent. A recent study by David Cutler, Mark McClellan, and Joseph Newhouse provides evidence that seems to confirm the relative importance of selective contracting.[36] These researchers examine medical claims data from a large employer that offered its employees a choice of several health plans, including HMOs and a standard indemnity plan. They focus on the costs of cardiovascular disease and find that medical costs were substantially lower in HMOs than in the indemnity plan, which they attribute to HMOs paying lower prices rather than HMO patients receiving fewer services.

The tempting conclusion from this study is that, at least in the case of patients with cardiovascular disease, managed care has largely failed to live up to its promise of reducing moral hazard and demand inducement. Rather, MCOs reduce costs by lowering payments to providers without eliminating wasteful utilization. There is a more favorable interpretation of the findings. Perhaps providers deliver the same level of care to all their patients but adjust that level up or down according to their patient mix. Providers who have many indemnity patients may deliver more services to all their patients. But as their mix moves toward managed care, they provide fewer services. Most doctors with whom I have spoken believe that this is an accurate description of how they conduct their own practices. If this is the behavior underlying the data in Cutler, McClellan, and Newhouse's study, then perhaps MCO strategies such as changing incentives and UR do make a difference.

Cutler, McClellan, and Newhouse examine cardiovascular disease, which may be life-threatening. Ann Barry Flood et al. examine resource utilization of HMO and indemnity patients with a variety of less severe diseases, including ear infections and eczema.[37] Working with data from a single medical clinic that treats both types of patients, these researchers find that patients with very minor or very severe conditions receive comparable services regardless of insurance. But moderately ill HMO patients receive fewer services, in large part because the HMOs in question use financial incentives to discourage patients and their PCPs from seeking the help of specialists. It seems that in this case, incentives do matter after all.

Managed Care and the Health Care Quadrilemma

If Burton Weisbrod's characterization of the health care quadrilemma is correct, then cost savings resulting from either lower prices or reductions in utilization may be only the tip of the iceberg. According to the quadrilemma, managed care will reduce incentives for providers to use new technologies. This, in turn, will change the incentives facing R&D firms. In the long run, R&D firms may introduce more cost-reducing technologies, with profound implications for the future cost and quality of care.

Several studies have confirmed one critical link in the quadrilemma, namely, that managed care is affecting both the use and the rate of adoption of new medical technologies. In the most comprehensive study to date, David Cutler and Louise Sheiner find that the rate of adoption of eighteen costly medical technologies, including angioplasty, radioisotope implants, Positron-emission tomography (PET) scanners, and bone marrow transplants, is lower in states that have high HMO penetration.[38] Using more detailed data on hospitals and MCOs, Cutler and Mark McClellan confirm these findings for angioplasty, and Michael Chernew, A. Mark Fendrick, and Richard Hirth confirm them for laparoscopic cholecystectomy.[39] In an interesting case study of what happened in Madison, Wisconsin, after legislation forced most employees into MCOs, Stephen Hill and Barbara Wolfe identify the microlevel dynamics associated with these reductions. Prior to the legislation, hospitals in Madison frequently engaged in a medical arms race, with much duplication of technology.[40] After the legislation and the subsequent growth of MCOs, the hospitals entered into several joint ventures for technologies such as lithotripters. Through reductions in the acquisition and use of costly technologies, these hospitals have dramatically reduced their costs.

If Weisbrod is right, the shifting demands for new technologies should affect medical research and development. Weisbrod and I conducted a survey of medical R&D firms to try to pin down some of these effects. The vice presidents of medical R&D whom we surveyed reported that their research projects have an increasing focus on cost containment, but they also reported that their projects have a growing potential to improve health. If the responses are accurate, this is exciting news for patients. But Weisbrod and I cannot be sure that these changes are due to incentives rather than scientific advances such as gene therapy. Future researchers will require more detailed information about individual medical R&D projects before the full implications of managed care, as played out through the quadrilemma, are identified.

Effects of Managed Care on Quality

There is no reason to conclude, based on theory alone, that quality must suffer under managed care. Physicians in the traditional health economy certainly provided more services than do those under managed care, but as we have learned from demand inducement, more care is not necessarily better care. Physicians in the traditional health economy also had complete decision-making authority, but as we have learned from medical practice variations, unfettered physician decision making is not necessarily better decision making. The effect of managed care on quality is, necessarily, an empirical matter. Despite widespread perceptions that managed care has harmed quality, the evidence to date is decidedly ambiguous.

Most surveys show that HMO enrollees and indemnity insurance enrollees are about equally satisfied with the quality of care in their plans.[41] But most enrollees are healthy most of the time, and critics point out that what really matters is the satisfaction of those who fall ill. Some surveys account for this, asking enrollees about the quality of their care while they were sick. Again, there are usually no meaningful differences.

Of course, survey responses can be misleading. Most patients lack the expertise to determine if they are receiving quality care. It is more meaningful to examine outcomes, such as mortality, morbidity, and functional status (e.g., whether the patient was able to resume a normal lifestyle). Summarizing this research is risky, because there are new studies of MCO quality every month. It is possible that by the time this book is published, the findings cited herein may be obsolete. But this seems unlikely. Each month's new studies generally confirm what many have already concluded, namely, that the quality of care in MCOs is comparable to that under traditional indemnity insurance.

In a 1996 study, Fred Hellinger reviews the published literature on HMO quality and concludes that there were few measurable differences between managed care and indemnity insurance on a variety of outcome measures.[42] Robert Miller and Harold Luft reach similar conclusions in their review of thirty-five studies published between 1993 and 1997. Miller and Luft sum up their findings as follows: "Fears that HMOs uniformly lead to worse quality of care are not supported by the evidence. . . . Hopes that HMOs would improve overall quality also are not supported."[43] More recent studies continue to refute the conventional wisdom that quality of care is worse in MCOs. A 1998 Johns Hopkins University review of the research on cardiovascular care, for example, concludes that "the HMOs studied provided as good, and in some cases better, quality than the non-HMO settings studied."[44]

Some studies find that HMOs deliver superior quality. The Dartmouth research team that found unacceptably low mammography and colon cancer screening rates among the general Medicare population also found that the rates were much higher among Medicare patients enrolled in HMOs. The results of higher screening rates are tangible: patients who belong to HMOs were more likely to obtain an early diagnosis of their breast cancer than were non-HMO Medicare patients. A Harvard research team found that heart attack patients covered by Medicare HMOs received slightly better care than did similar patients with traditional HMO coverage.[45] Another recent study found that nursing home residents enrolled in HMOs received higher quality care than non-HMO residents, perhaps because they have frequent contact with allied medical personnel such as nurse-practitioners.[46]

Not all the evidence on HMO quality is favorable. Both Hellinger and Miller and Luft find some evidence that low-income and Medicare patients with chronic conditions fared worse in HMOs. A more recent study, published by the *Journal of the American Medical Association*, found that low-income and Medicare patients enrolled in HMOs for four years or more had lower self-reported health status.[47]

Overall, the evidence suggests that HMOs score higher on some dimensions of quality and lower on others, and on many other dimensions quality is about even. A spate of research in progress appears likely to reach the same conclusions. The mixed empirical evidence belies the many complaints about HMOs. Physicians complain the loudest, apparently unwilling to accept even the possibility of reduced quality in exchange for $300 billion in annual savings. Perhaps conditioned by the complaints of their physicians, patients are complaining as well. In the aforementioned study of quality in nursing homes, even though HMO enrollees received demonstrably higher quality care, they believed that they were receiving lower quality care. Why the disconnect between perception and reality? I believe that one important reason is that patients in HMOs feel they lack adequate access to physicians. Patients equate access to physicians with quality, regardless of whether the access is to needed services or just a source of comfort, with no other health benefit. At the same time, patients appear to take the services offered by HMOs for granted and do not realize that if they were not in an HMO they might not receive the needed mammography or colon cancer screen. Unless and until consumers take a more sophisticated view of quality, HMOs will necessarily look bad in comparison with traditional fee-for-service medicine.

Effects on Trust

While the evidence of the effects of managed care on quality is ambiguous, the evidence of its effects on trust is clear. Studies repeatedly show that while most Americans continue to trust their physicians, they do not trust MCOs. In a recent survey conducted jointly by the Henry Kaiser Family Foundation, Harvard University, and Princeton Research Associates, only 30 percent of respondents enrolled in managed care trusted their plans to "do the right thing for their care," versus 55 percent enrolled in traditional plans.[48] In an annual survey conducted by Louis Harris and Associates for over thirty years, the percentage of respondents indicating that they have "hardly any" confidence in medicine rose from an average of 6 percent between 1966 and 1975, to 12 percent between 1976 and 1986, and to 18 percent between 1987 and 1997. Another recent study published in the *Journal of the American Medical Association* finds that fewer than 30 percent of patients trust their HMOs to control costs without adversely affecting quality.[49]

These findings of a general distrust in managed care often are at odds with how patients feel about their own HMO. Indeed, even though enrollees usually report high satisfaction with the quality of care provided by their own HMO, the majority of respondents to a 1997 Kaiser/Harvard/ Princeton survey report that HMOs decrease the quality of health care. At the same time, respondents to the same survey do not believe that HMOs have helped lower medical costs.

What is behind this extraordinary level of discontent? MCOs score poorly on all three of Mechanic's dimensions of trust. Patients do not trust in the compassion of MCOs. Most MCOs are for-profit, and many rely on financial incentives to change provider behavior. Patients are skeptical of this mixing of dollars with medicine. Nor do patients trust the competence of MCOs. Occasional newspaper accounts of MCO "horror stories" reinforce criticism by the medical profession and cause patients to question the quality of care, even if the systematic research says otherwise and their own experiences are generally favorable. Patients also are concerned that aggressive intervention by MCOs might limit the ability of their doctors to control and coordinate the resources necessary to delivery quality care. In some cases, patients who are unable to see their preferred specialist blame their PCP along with their MCO, further eroding trust in the health care system.[50]

From Marcus Welby to Managed Care

When television's *Marcus Welby, M.D.*, aired in the 1960s, Americans placed great trust in their health care system. Costs were low but were beginning their rapid ascent. Americans believed that they were getting high-quality care, though they really could not tell. In the ensuing thirty years, the health economy has evolved from Marcus Welby medicine to managed care. MCOs certainly obtain better prices from providers than patients could on their own. There is even evidence that MCOs limit moral hazard utilization and demand inducement, while forcing providers to rationalize the adoption and use of costly technologies. As a result, Americans in the past decade have enjoyed a respite from double-digit health care cost increases. But America's trust in the health economy has eroded, and patients still do not know much about quality.

Where is the health economy headed? Managed care has introduced a previously unseen market discipline to insurers and providers. As described in the next three chapters, they have responded with a range of strategies. As we will see, some of these strategies threaten to undermine managed care, but a few hold out the promise of doing what neither Marcus Welby medicine nor managed care as currently executed has been able to do: assure patients high quality at a reasonable cost. If these strategies succeed, America's trust in the health economy may be restored, and such trust will be based on facts rather than blind faith. For the first time, patients may actually know something about quality, and the quality they receive will be very good indeed.

Part Two

THE MODERN HEALTH ECONOMY

CHAPTER 5

The Business of Health Care

HEALTH CARE in the United States is a trillion-dollar industry. Even small players in the industry are fairly large by the standards of many other industries. A modest group practice of five physicians can generate revenues of $3 million or more annually (more than the annual revenue of a typical McDonald's franchise). A community hospital can generate revenues of $100 million (more than the annual revenue of some major-league baseball teams), and some teaching hospitals have revenues exceeding $500 million annually (roughly twice the 1999 net revenue of the Internet auction site eBay). Increasingly, the managers of these large enterprises have degrees from the nation's top business schools, and many were successful business leaders in other industries before coming to health care. To help these managers, huge support industries have emerged in health care marketing, accounting, consulting, and investment banking. At the same time, the nation's largest employers have hired expert benefits managers to oversee their multi-million-dollar expenditures for health insurance. With so much emphasis on business, there seems to be little room for Marcus Welby in the modern health economy.

The injection of business principles into the health economy has many virtues, however. Through their MCOs, patients can purchase health care services at discount prices. To stay competitive, providers constantly seek to reduce costs and boost quality. But the downside of turning medicine into a business is inescapable. The reasons offered by Kenneth Arrow for organizing the health economy around professional physician-agents and nonprofit hospitals have not disappeared. It remains difficult for patients to measure the performance of their providers. Quality is still a matter of trust. In the rest of this book, I explore what patients have gained and lost in the modern health economy and identify what patients and providers must do to take full advantage of the promise of managed care.

IT STARTS WITH EMPLOYERS

Nowadays, before a doctor can select a treatment, the health plan must select the doctor. But even before that, the employer must select the health plan.[1] By selecting the plan, the employer becomes an agent for its employees/During the era of Marcus Welby medicine, employer-agents had little to do. Competing insurance plans were virtually identical, offering indemnity coverage with unlimited access to physicians and hospitals. Employers selected a plan mainly on the basis of price and customer service, where good service was taken to mean prompt and accurate payment of bills.

When employers first turned to MCOs to hold down health care costs, they knew little about them and so relied on independent benefits consultants to sort out their choices. When many of these consultants seemed to know less about managed care than did their clients, some employers took it upon themselves to develop expertise in health plan selection. They beefed up the health insurance section of their benefits departments and gave the same consideration to the purchase of health insurance as they did to the procurement of other key productive inputs. By the 1990s, large employers were adopting what the United States General Accounting Office described as an "active purchasing strategy, . . . a systematic way of identifying and offering a mix of health care options that meet a purchaser's expectations in terms of access, quality, and price."[2]

Some employers choose a single plan for their employees. By being so selective, these employers reduce the costs of managing benefits and can sometimes obtain favorable premiums. Employees at these firms depend on their employer to select the plan that best balances access, quality, and price. Larger employers usually give their employees a choice of plan, letting them select the one that best meets their needs. These employers obtain favorable rates by only offering a few plans, and the competition that results from employee choice further holds down rates. Because they both have a say in plan selection, employers and employees are jointly responsible for balancing access, quality, and price.

Whose Side Are Employers On?

Whether offering a single plan or a menu of plans, employers shoulder a significant responsibility. If they care about MCO quality, MCOs will have to provide it. If they ignore quality, MCOs might be able to ignore it as well. It is not obvious whether employers will give remotely the same consideration to quality as their employees would like. The fact that employers offer insurance at all is a good sign. Economists have noted that one of the most cost-effective ways for employers to attract and retain good employees is to offer health insurance. Most workers would find it fairly expensive to purchase insurance on their own. Not only is it costly for insurers to write individual policies, but insurers prefer selling to employer groups, which tend to have stable health care risks. In addition, employees who obtain insurance through work get tax advantages not normally available to individuals who purchase insurance on their own. Thus, it is natural for employees to look to their employers for insurance coverage.

In a perfect world, employers would offer the health insurance plan that employees would have purchased on their own, presumably one that does not sacrifice quality just to save a few dollars. Employers would then adjust wages up or down according to the price of the plan. In the real world, it must be very tempting for employers to offer the lowest cost plan regardless of its quality. After all, most employees pay very little attention to elements of plan design that most affect the cost-quality trade-off—use of incentives, stringency of UR, and so forth. Small, struggling employers often do select the cheapest plans. (Salespeople at one well-regarded HMO in Illinois tell me that they have all but given up selling to small employers because they cannot compete on price.) But larger firms tend to be more careful shoppers, and their benefits managers usually scrutinize all aspects of plan design before selecting a plan. As will be described in Chapter 7, a few big firms have taken bold steps to promote higher MCO quality. The hope is that enough employers care about quality to put MCOs on notice: any MCO that focuses on cost and totally disregards quality will be no better than a niche player in its market.

HOW PROVIDERS COPE WITH MANAGED CARE

MCOs are under growing pressure from employers to reduce costs while maintaining or boosting quality. Through selective contracting, MCOs are placing the same pressures on providers. In this way, providers are feeling the heat from competition and are coming face-to-face with the business side of medicine. This has brought many positive (and some not so positive) changes to the U.S. health economy.

Even before the huge growth in managed care in the 1990s, Medicare's Prospective Payment System had already given hospitals reason to be concerned about their costs. Hospitals initially reacted to the PPS by curtailing services—cutting lengths of stay, reducing inpatient testing, and laying off staff. The results were immediately evident: 1983–85 saw the lowest increase in hospital costs in decades. Moreover, there is no evidence that quality suffered. Enthoven's conjecture about flat-of-the-curve medicine seemed to be right.

Medicare took advantage of these cost reductions (or, more accurately, reductions in the rate of growth of costs) by cutting the amount it paid to hospitals for inpatient care. This kicked off a cycle in which hospitals took steps to reduce inpatient costs, Medicare reduced payments, hospitals cut costs further, and so forth. Soon, MCOs joined in the price-cutting, further pressuring hospitals to reduce costs. Pushed by these financial incentives and aided by improvements in surgical techniques and anesthetics, hospitals responded by providing more outpatient care. In 1984, 28 percent of all surgeries performed at community hospitals were done on an outpatient basis. By 1996, the figure had jumped to 59 percent, and this does not account for surgeries performed at freestanding surgery centers. Today, most patients who undergo hernia repair, diagnostic colonoscopies, tonsillectomies, cataract extractions, and CT scans, to name just a few procedures, are treated as outpatients.

To further curtail costs, many hospitals have cut back on uncompensated care, and many teaching hospitals have cut back on research.[3] As hospital resources continue to dwindle, the public will have to either accept these cutbacks or find a way to avoid them through a combination of tax-subsidized government programs and private sector initiatives. This is not necessarily a bad thing. Prior to managed care, hospitals subsidized research and uncompensated care "in secret," through the high prices they charged under patient-driven competition. Without the secret subsidies, taxpayers will have an opportunity to decide how much they really want to spend on research and uncompensated care.

Layoffs, shifts to outpatient care, and reductions in research and uncompensated care are the low-hanging fruit of cost containment. A health care manager "merely" has to take a pen to a budget, and expenditures fall. But these shortcuts to savings can only go so far. The big savings, and the greatest value in the face of competition, come from gains in efficiency. In their quest for efficiency, providers have relied on strategies common throughout business—continuous quality improvement and reengineering. Through these strategies, providers are eliminating some of the fat that accumulated in the traditional health economy.

Cutting Costs While Boosting Quality: CQI

During the 1980s, health care providers joined the continuous quality improvement (CQI) movement that was sweeping the corporate world. Developed by American business educators but perfected by Japanese automotive and electronics firms, CQI reduces costs by eliminating defects in production processes. It stands to reason that production defects—whether they occur in the production of a car or in the treatment of an illness—can simultaneously reduce quality and increase costs. The goal of every CQI program is "zero defects." CQI became popular in the United States in the 1980s, especially when companies such as Ford and Motorola received favorable publicity for using it to match or even surpass the efficiencies of their Japanese rivals.

By the late 1980s, most hospitals expressed an interest in CQI, and the majority had launched CQI programs by 1992. By 1997, nearly all hospitals reported using the approach, with many spending hundreds of thousands of dollars annually on their CQI efforts. Hospital CQI programs vary from sending a few staff to an off-site seminar to hiring personnel trained in CQI or even creating new departments charged with implementing CQI programs. Although there is no hard evidence, it seems likely that many other health care organizations, including larger physician groups, have also jumped on the CQI bandwagon.

Many types of programs fall under the CQI umbrella. As one example, a urology group sought to improve the quality and reduce the cost of care for prostate cancer patients.[4] The group developed a flowchart showing all the steps in the medical care process, before, during, and after the hospital stay. The flowchart enabled the group to identify factors associated with delayed recovery, such as improper and costly surgical techniques (e.g., the use of surgical staples), inadequate feeding, and misuse of drugs and blood supplies. The group also reorganized nurse staffing and identified two physicians with poor outcomes who underwent subsequent retraining. It was estimated that as a result of these changes, the total cost of care fell by 25 percent.

In a 1998 publication, a team led by Stephen Shortell reviews the lengthy academic literature on CQI and finds over fifty studies like the prostate study just mentioned.[5] Shortell's team finds that the majority of studies presented evidence favorable to CQI, including reduced lengths of stay, lower charges, lower costs, and reduced mortality. They point out that in virtually all of these studies, the participants chose to implement CQI themselves, leaving open the possibility of selection bias. (Selection bias would creep in if, for example, providers who implemented CQI tended to have unusually high costs and would have realized some savings even if they did not implement CQI.) They find only two randomized clinical trials of CQI, neither one of which could attribute any changes in costs or outcomes to CQI. Despite widespread acceptance by providers, the evidence on the effectiveness of CQI is not overwhelming.

Practice Guidelines and Disease Management: Striving for Efficiency

Health care providers have borrowed another cost containment strategy from the corporate world: reengineering. Whereas CQI focuses on eliminating mistakes in existing processes, reengineering introduces new processes. Reengineering is a broad concept that encompasses a wide range of practices, from adopting software for scheduling patients in the operating room to consolidating of departments that are overstaffed. Perhaps because the definition of reengineering is so vague, hospitals that have used the strategy report little improvement in their financial performance, and the number of hospitals introducing additional reengineering programs has fallen precipitously in the past few years. (According to one report, 144 hospitals started reengineering programs in 1995, but only 10 did so in 1997.)

Thus far, reengineering has often been little more than a gussied-up way to describe normal business practices. The future of reengineering lies in finding new ways to deliver medical care, as exemplified by treatment guidelines and disease management programs. These two terms are often used interchangeably, but their differences are worth noting. Providers use *treatment guidelines* to improve performance during discrete medical episodes such as a hospital stay or visit to a clinic. *Disease management*, which is broader than treatment guidelines, provides direction for coordinating the delivery of health care resources throughout the life cycle of disease, from prevention and diagnosis through treatment and recovery.

Like utilization review, treatment guidelines and disease management programs are a direct response to medical practice variations. Also like UR, they are based on careful examination of the research literature on treatment efficacy. But unlike UR, they have not been unilaterally imposed by MCOs. While some MCOs do impose some treatment guidelines and disease management programs on providers, it is more common for providers to adopt them voluntarily. This may explain why providers have been so much more receptive to guidelines and disease management than they have been to UR. Even so, providers would have been unlikely to so thoroughly embrace them were it not for market pressures to reduce costs and improve quality.

Hospitals have guidelines for treating a wide range of diseases, from AIDS to varicose veins. Guidelines typically provide the medical staff with detailed day-by-day instructions for testing, nursing, surgery (if appropriate), rehabilitation, and discharge planning. The ordering of tests and other medical services becomes systematized according to the precepts of the guidelines. For example, the federally funded Steering Committee on Clinical Practice Guidelines for the Care and Treatment of Breast Cancer recently published treatment guidelines for women with stage II breast cancer, which include specific recommendations for chemotherapy.[6]

While most hospitals (and virtually all other providers) lack the resources to develop their own guidelines from scratch, there is no shortage of independently developed guidelines to choose from and build on. A 1993 study finds that thirty commissions and eighty professional societies already were involved in developing guidelines.[7] By 1994, the American Medical Association had collected over sixteen hundred guidelines, and there undoubtedly have been thousands more developed since then. With so many guidelines, there are bound to be inconsistencies, which becomes more problematic when the MCO guideline says "do not treat" and the provider guideline says "treat." One health care executive, commenting about the proliferation of guidelines, derisively described them as "the octopus of managed care."[8] With so many guidelines to choose from, physicians have a difficult time keeping up. Many advocates of guidelines, such as Alan Hillman of the University of Pennsylvania, are optimistic that MCOs can coordinate their guidelines with hospitals, creating a small number of guidelines that are "seamless to the provider and patient."[9]

The federal Agency for Healthcare Research and Quality has been a major catalyst for the development of disease management protocols.[10] Starting in the 1980s, the agency funded patient outcome research teams or PORTs, to review the available evidence on efficacy and recommend treatment norms for dozens of diseases, including ischemic heart disease, non-insulin-dependent diabetes mellitus, cataracts, and prostate cancer. For example, in 1998 the *Schizoprenia Bulletin* published the final report of the schizoprenia PORT, which issued recommendations on drug therapy, psychological interventions, rehabilitation, and community treatment. In 1997, the *Archives of Internal Medicine* reported interim results from the pneumonia PORT, which found that "the availability of outpatient intravenous antimicrobial therapy and home nursing care would allow for outpatient care for a larger proportion of low-risk patients who are hospitalized."[11] In the last two years, the AHRQ played a supportive role in developing disease management programs. Rather than continue to develop its own programs, it will increasingly provide the data and literature reviews necessary for private sector organizations to do the work.

Providers, especially teaching hospitals, have also developed disease management programs. They often incorporate information from the PORTS, as well as their own research, to develop unique programs. One can find some of these programs on the Internet, on diseases ranging from obstructive lung disease (a Stanford University site) and vascular disease (Montefiore Medical Center) to Huntington's disease (Baylor College of Medicine) and AIDS (the International Assocation of Physicians in AIDS care). A recent survey of twenty-five health care organizations, including HMOs, indemnity insurers, and physician groups, finds that every one was involved in some kind of treatment guideline or disease management program.[12] Patients and providers should expect to see more Web sites as these programs mature and providers seek to share their findings.

Some businesses see disease management as an opportunity to make a profit. Most major health care consulting firms have their own disease management practices and sell their findings to MCOs and providers. Pharmaceutical companies have also developed disease management programs centered around their products. During the 1990s, three companies—Merck, Eli Lilly, and SmithKline—spent billions of dollars to acquire pharmacy benefits management firms (PBMs), in large part to acquire data that could help them develop disease management programs. Recent mergers of giant MCOs are also motivated by the desire to assemble large utilization databases. Providers have not been especially eager to use the programs developed by drug makers and MCOs, however, and Lilly and SmithKline recently took billion-dollar losses when they sold their PBM divisions.

Blueprints for Care

Treatment guidelines and disease management programs are like blueprints for the provision of medical care. Blueprints have their advantages. In home building, they assure that all the building parts are exactly the right size and fit together perfectly, that nothing is left out, and that nothing is done to excess. The same is true in medicine, where the treatment guidelines and disease management "blueprints" assure the proper timing of all required services while avoiding duplication and waste. In theory, guidelines within the hospital can cut down on the ordering of tests, demands on nursing time, and misuse of medications. Guidelines can facilitate scheduling of the operating room, intensive care, and discharge planning. In theory, disease management can help providers identify medical problems in their earliest stages and prescribe the most cost-effective therapies. Guidelines and disease management are potentially far more effective in eliminating inappropriate variations in medical practice than UR, which is largely limited to simple decisions about the need for surgery and the appropriate length of inpatient stay.

Of course, blueprints have their disadvantages. Blueprints drawn up for a large-scale housing development do not meet the needs of every homeowner, and many home buyers insist on customization. In medicine, blueprints do not meet the needs of every patient, whose idiosyncratic needs may justify "customization" of the medical care process. In part because providers are concerned about idiosyncracies, and in part because guidelines are so new, provider compliance with guidelines is usually voluntary. For example, insurers belonging to the Colorado Cooperative for Health Insurance Purchasing report guidelines for diabetes, colorectal screening, childhood immunizations, and prenatal care, and even send their providers reports showing how they compare with norms.[13] But they do not punish providers who depart from norms. This permits providers to try to strike a balance between adhering to the blueprints for the sake of following desired norms and departing from the blueprints to meet the idiosyncratic needs of patients. Providers prefer this to UR-type programs that mandate that they follow norms.

Many physicians are even skeptical about voluntary guidelines and disease management. They know that the quality of blueprints depends on the knowledge and motivations of the individuals who design them. As a result, they often distrust guidelines and disease management programs developed by "outsiders" to the medical community, especially pharmaceutical companies (which are often perceived as pushing their products rather than selling treatments). At the same time, physicians recognize that blueprints are only as good as the data used to create them, and there is ample room for improving health care data, as I will discuss later.

While there is a rich literature showing how various guidelines and disease management programs can change physician behavior, there is little systematic evidence that guidelines and disease management actually improve outcomes or reduce costs. Neither providers nor MCOs can state with certainty that any particular guideline will be successful until they try to implement it. Nor do they know whether voluntary compliance is preferred to mandated compliance. In the absence of empirical evaluations of guidelines and disease management, physicians who are wedded to a particular way of treating patients have an excuse not to follow the blueprints. This creates a chicken-or-egg problem for the blueprints. A guideline that seems appropriate in theory may fail to generate interest among physicians, thereby making it difficult to develop empirical evidence to support the guideline, thereby giving physicians an excuse not to follow it, and so forth. Even so, virtually all health care managers are banking on these strategies to become more efficient. A key managerial challenge will be to find ways to effectively implement and administer the programs, both to enlist the support of skeptical physicians and to permit them to strike the balance between norms and idiosyncracies.

A Victory for Managed Care

Even if CQI, treatment guidelines, and disease management turn out to be relatively ineffective, the exciting lesson to be learned from their development is that managed care has forced providers to think about efficiency. This is a tremendous victory for managed care. It seems doubtful that managers would be pursuing these innovative strategies were it not for the competitive pressures of the marketplace. Indeed, these strategies are far less common among health care providers outside the United States, where cost containment pressure comes from regulation rather than from the market. Contrast the United States, where these strategies have been undertaken for well over a decade, with Great Britain. One of the leading

British medical journals, the *Lancet*, described the 1999 formation of a government agency to develop guidelines in England as a "quiet revolution."[14] That revolution is a way of life for U.S. health care providers.

The U.S. experience suggests that competition is a powerful force for innovation in health care delivery. Perhaps this reflects the view, unique to the United States, that the provision of health care is a business, so that health care managers frequently look to other businesses for fresh ways to improve the performance of their organizations. (It is noteworthy that prior to the growth of managed care, health care managers were called *administrators*, a term that is still common in other nations.) Even if today's health care managers find that CQI, treatment guidelines, and disease management programs ultimately fail to live up to their promise, they will surely pursue other routes to efficiency. Such are the benefits of a competitive market.

MAXIMIZING REVENUES

Whether or not providers successfully reduce costs, they can also cope with competitive pressures by boosting their revenues. Providers who are "in demand" thrive by raising their prices well above their costs. More than any other providers, hospitals have made substantial investments in marketing, so they can evaluate their competitive position, attempt to differentiate themselves from the crowd, and price accordingly.

A look at the makeup of hospital networks assembled by MCOs reveals the types of hospitals that providers look for.[15] Hospital networks invariably include at least one local teaching hospital, as well as community hospitals from all geographic areas of the local market.[16] The network selected by any given employer is also sure to include the hospital at which the CEO's physician has admitting privileges. In other words, employers want to give their employees (and themselves) access to both local hospitals and at least one tertiary care hospital. The end result is that most networks include most local hospitals. Employers pay a price for having such broad networks. MCOs could negotiate lower prices if they were willing to exclude more hospitals from their networks. But employees want access, and employers are willing to pay the price to give it to them. The market forces the MCOs to oblige. This helps explain why MCO prices have crept up in the past few years as they have expanded their networks to offer what the market demands.

Teaching status, favorable locations, and a well-connected medical staff are not the only ways for hospitals to add value to a network. Hospitals believe that they can catch the attention of employees, and achieve "must include" status in networks, by establishing "centers of excellence."

Hospitals have established such centers for fertility, heart disease, sports medicine, holistic medicine, substance abuse, and even male reproductive health. Sometimes a hospital slaps the "center" label on an existing program and hopes that clever advertisements will help it stand out. In other cases, hospitals make large investments to build a competency in the clinical area by recruiting leading physicians and providing the necessary technological and human resources to provide state-of-the-art treatment. Centers of excellence enable hospitals to develop a critical mass of expertise and experience needed to move down the learning curve and provide better quality.

The emergence of centers of excellence harkens back to the days of facilities planning. One of the goals of the National Health Planning and Resources Development Act of 1974 was to create regional referral centers that specialize in certain services: there was to be one center for heart surgery, another for diabetes, and so forth. Because certificate-of-need enforcement was so ineffectual, such centers did not emerge. Now market forces seem to be moving hospitals in the same direction, but consumers have not flocked to these centers in any great numbers (perhaps because they perceive them to be marketing ploys rather than quality enhancements), and most hospitals continue to provide most kinds of treatment. The growth of centers of excellence has done little thus far to concentrate care in a smaller number of "excellent" facilities.

In fact, the slow development of centers of excellence provides an example of how government planning in other nations has been more effective than market forces in the United States. In many other nations, including Canada, regional referral centers are common. However, there is no evidence that quality at these referral centers is higher than at the many competing providers in the United States.

Playing Reimbursement Games

During the regulatory decade of the 1970s, hospitals learned that they could increase revenues by responding creatively to reimbursement rules. This lesson has not been lost, as hospitals continue to play reimbursement games, particularly in the Medicare Prospective Payment System. Upcoding, first mentioned in Chapter 3, provides a good example. There is often a large gray area between diagnosis-related groups, so that hospitals can maximize reimbursements by classifying patients into more remunerative groups. In recent years, HCFA has cracked down on hospitals that it believed were excessively exploiting the ambiguities in DRG coding. In a well-publicized example, HCFA accused Columbia/HCA hospitals of inconsistent diagnostic coding, with the implication that the inconsistencies facilitated upcoding. HCFA subsequently leveled similar charges against several nonprofit hospitals, showing that for-profits do not have a monopoly on bending the rules. Because HCFA reduces its DRG payments across the board to account for upcoding, hospitals may feel that they have to upcode; otherwise, they would receive lower reimbursements than their less scrupulous rivals. Unfortunately, upcoding distorts medical records, generating diagnoses that maximize reimbursements rather than reflect the patient's health.

Many believe that the zeal to reduce inpatient utilization that started with Medicare's PPS and continues with private sector UR has encouraged another form of gamesmanship called *unbundling*. Services that were once provided during the course of a single hospitalization are now provided in a host of settings. A freestanding diagnostic facility may provide the initial workup. After a brief hospital stay, the patient may be transferred for recovery in a subacute ward and discharged under the supervision of a home health care nurse, with subsequent follow-up visits to hospital clinics. Through such unbundling, providers augment the DRG-based hospital bill with bills for each outpatient service. In a particularly vexatious variation on this strategy, hospitals (for-profits and nonprofits alike) convert inpatient wards into skilled nursing facilities (SNFs). HCFA pays a fixed daily rate for care in SNFs. Hospitals that discharge patients to their own SNFs, rather than keep them as inpatients, receive the flat fee for the inpatient stay *and* a daily SNF payment. The patient is no better off (and may be worse off for the inconvenience), but the hospital gets more revenue.

Upcoding, unbundling, and other strategies to maximize reimbursements rarely threaten our health, though they do rob our purses. They also confirm the importance of incentives for hospitals, whether the health economy is regulated or driven by competition, and whether the hospitals are investor-owned or nonprofits.

THE BUSINESS OF BEING A PHYSICIAN

From my own experience, it seems that one can do a pretty good job of predicting how a physician feels about managed care, especially HMOs, just by knowing his or her age. Physicians over age fifty-five spent most of their careers practicing Marcus Welby medicine. They are reasonably wealthy and can almost disregard the changes taking place around them. Older physicians disproportionately concentrate their practice on non-HMO Medicare patients and the dwindling number of patients with private, indemnity insurance.[17] They may not like HMOs, but they have managed to ignore them. Physicians between the ages of forty and fifty-five entered medical school before the rise of managed care. They are now practicing medicine in an environment that is far different than what they expected at the start of their careers. They are too young to turn a blind eye to the changes, but they are unhappy about having to accommodate HMOs, and they tend to be the most vocal opponents of managed care. Younger physicians knew about managed care when they entered medical school and were ready to meet the challenges upon graduation. In disproportionate numbers, young physicians have introduced information and accounting systems to their practices, developed treatment guidelines and disease management programs, joined group practices and newer organizational arrangements such as physician-hospital organizations, and welcomed contracts with HMOs.

Many physicians have embraced the business side of medicine. Nowhere is this more apparent than in ongoing educational programs. Not long ago, a physician's ongoing education consisted of attending seminars on the latest clinical developments and reading medical journals. Now, it is not unusual for physicians to attend management seminars and read medical management journals with articles like "Developing a Medical Practice Mission Statement," "Do You Need an Office Manager or an Office Administrator?" and "Managed Care Contracting." A small but growing number of young physicians have taken the need for management training seriously and are pursuing M.B.A. degrees either concurrently with or after their M.D. training. The ongoing business education of physicians is a rapidly growing industry.

Physician Practice Management

Despite management journals and business courses, the management skills of most physicians have not kept pace with the demands made by managed care for business expertise. A primary problem in this regard is that most physicians practice either on their own or in small groups and cannot afford the time and money to develop, adopt, and master CQI programs, clinical guidelines, cost-accounting systems, and other practices necessary to thrive under managed care.

Unable to cope with the business of medicine, many physicians have sought help from professional managers. Physicians have always relied on office managers to handle routine business affairs, including hiring, billing, and maintaining medical records. With the growth of managed care, and the complexities involved in handling claims, obtaining UR approval, and dealing with a myriad of reimbursement rules, physicians have hired many more nonmedical personnel, and the clerical staff of a small physician group can outnumber the medical staff. In the past decade, many physicians have stopped trying to run the business side of their practice altogether and have sold their practice assets and a share of their practice revenue (usually 15 percent) to *physician practice management* (PPM) firms. In exchange, the PPMs take total control over the business side of the practice. MedPartners, once the nation's largest PPM, described its role this way: "We manage everything about a physician's practice . . . except the practice of medicine."

Roughly sixty thousand physicians (about 10 percent of all M.D.'s) have affiliations with PPMs. In their promotional literature, PPMs boast about their "partnerships" with physicians. But most affiliated physicians are not seeking new partners so much as they are seeking help. Physicians need financial capital to acquire new equipment; they want to expand their offices to accommodate more nurses and nurse-practitioners, so they can handle the bigger caseloads required for a prosperous MCO practice; they need information systems to handle complex billing and medical records keeping; they need help negotiating with MCOs; they want to purchase supplies at the lowest possible prices. PPMs help physicians do all these things.

Physicians obviously have much to gain by turning to PPMs for management expertise. Even so, PPMs have failed to live up to their own investors' expectations. In late 1998, MedPartners announced that it was divesting its PPM business, concentrating instead on pharmacy benefits management. This followed a dismal performance on Wall Street that also hit other PPMs, including PhyCor and Pediatrix. One reason that PPMs like MedPartners failed to meet Wall Street's expectations is that they grew too rapidly, paying too much to purchase too many practices. MedPartners was especially set back when it paid premium prices to acquire smaller PPMs but failed to create additional value. PPMs also learned a hard lesson about incentives. In many cases, physicians who sold their practices did not work as hard as they did when they were their own bosses. In fact, it seems likely that the physicians who sold out to PPMs were the ones who most wanted to curtail their practices anyway. These incentive problems loom large over the PPM market. Unless there is a creative solution, PPMs may fail to achieve their goal (as stated by PhyCor in its Web site): "To create, with physicians, the best value in medical care for our communities."

PHARMACY BENEFITS MANAGEMENT

Managed care came to pharmaceuticals in the late 1980s, when pharmacy benefits management firms such as Medco, PCS Health Systems, Diversified Pharmaceutical Services (DPS), Express Scripts, and Value Rx successfully injected price competition into the market. Before PBMs, there was not much price competition among pharmaceutical firms. A variety of factors—similar to those that embodied patient-driven competition among hospitals—enabled drug makers to set prices well in excess of their marginal costs. Most working Americans had insurance to foot the bill and thus were insensitive to price. Patients who lacked insurance usually purchased the drug prescribed by their physician. They rarely asked their physician or pharmacist for a less costly alternative, in part because they did not know if alternatives existed. Facing little pressure from consumers to lower prices (except, occasionally, when there were low-priced generic alternatives), drug makers avoided price competition. They plowed their high margins into R&D and marketing, usually with enough profit left over to reward shareholders with solid returns.

Like the hospital market in the early 1980s, the pharmaceutical market in the early 1990s was ripe for selective contracting. PBMs obtain discounts from drug makers in much the same way that MCOs obtain discounts from other medical providers—by promising higher market shares in exchange for lower prices. If anything, PBMs have been even more successful than MCOs in this regard, obtaining discounts of as much as 80 percent off of retail prices. This is mainly due to the fact that the cost of producing many drugs is just a small fraction of the retail price.

What the network is to an MCO, the formulary is to the PBM—the list of covered drugs. To assure that patients have access to all available drug therapies, a typical formulary includes at least one drug from all classes of therapeutically equivalent drugs. For example, the formulary will include at least one H_2-antagonist (antiulcer) medication, such as Zantac or Tagamet, and one calcium channel blocker, such as Calan or Norvasc. The formulary might exclude a branded drug if a generic version (e.g., cimetidine or verapamil) is available.

To motivate drug makers to offer steep discounts, PBMs must steer patients toward drugs on the formulary. This is a challenge. By and large, patients can only obtain the drug written by their physician on the prescription. Thus, PBMs must get physicians to write prescriptions for drugs on the formulary. To do this, they make sure that physicians know what drugs are on their formularies; all else being equal, physicians are inclined to prescribe these drugs to save their patients' money. PBMs also encourage pharmacists to identify off-formulary prescriptions. Some PBMs provide software to pharmacists, enabling them to easily identify these problematic prescriptions, the "guilty" physicians, and the "correct" alternative drugs. The PBM (or the pharmacist) then contacts the physician to request a change in prescription. Finally, most PBMs encourage patients to use "mail-order" pharmacy to purchase chronic medications. Patients may require dozens of refills of these drugs and stand to save hundreds of dollars if their physicians keep to the mail-order formulary.

By any business standard, pharmacy benefits management has been a tremendous success. In less than a decade, PBMs have achieved nearly 100 percent penetration in private health insurance. By aggressively working to change physician prescribing practices, they have delivered on the promise of volume for discounts. Pharmaceutical manufacturers have fought back by aggressively advertising their branded drugs, in the hope that patients will insist on receiving the advertised brand. This forces physicians to write prescriptions for the branded drugs regardless of whether they are on formulary, and it ultimately forces PBMs to include advertised drugs on the formulary or lose favor with patients.

Pharmacoeconomics

PBMs are profoundly affecting pharmaceutical R&D. As a result, discounting may be only a small part of the PBM legacy. Every year, pharmaceutical manufacturers must decide how they will spend their massive R&D budgets. They might emphasize scientifically novel drugs that promise to offer substantial new benefits to patients. Or they might emphasize "me-too" drugs that mimic the chemical and therapeutic properties of drugs already on the market. Whatever they choose, it will usually cost them $200 million or more to shepherd the drug through the FDA approval process. With the advent of PBMs, there is no guarantee that drug makers can charge enough to recover the costs of R&D for me-too drugs. However, they can still charge high prices for novel drugs that have no therapeutic equivalents. Because this is where the profits lie, drug makers are shifting their research efforts away from me-too drugs and toward more scientifically challenging "breakthrough" innovations. This represents an unexpected fringe benefit of the rise of managed care.

Thanks to a combination of market forces and scientific advances, there have been a number of pharmaceutical breakthroughs in the late 1990s. Drugs such as Viagra (for the treatment of male sexual dysfunction) and Lupron (for the treatment of prostate cancer) deliver benefits to patients who previously had few, if any, drug options. But these drugs come at a steep price. Treatments for many chronic diseases can cost thousands of dollars annually; one new drug, Cerezyme (for Gaucher's disease), costs $150,000 for a year's treatment. In the future, customized, genetically engineered drugs may routinely cost this much or more.

MCO expenditures for pharmaceuticals have been rising at over 10 percent annually and are a major factor behind recent growth in MCO premiums. It has become imperative for many MCOs to slow the growth of drug costs. One important result is that a growing number of MCOs are asking PBMs to evaluate cost-benefit ratios for all drugs to be added to formularies, even those that lack a therapeutic equivalent. Pharmacoeconomics researchers review existing research on cost-effectiveness and perform original research to determine whether costly new drugs might generate offsetting savings, perhaps by reducing the need for hospitalization or by enabling the patient to return to the workforce. Drug manufacturers have their own pharmacoeconomists who conduct research that (they hope) will convince PBMs to include their drugs on formularies.

Quality Adjusted Life Years

Building on academic research, pharmacoeconomists have developed a scale, such as the Quality Adjusted Life Year (QALY) scale and the Healthy Years Equivalent (HYE) scale, for quantifying the health benefits of different interventions. The QALY scale is best known. Based on surveys in which patients indicate their "preferences" for different health states, the QALY scale assigns a score between 0 and 1 to every health condition, where death is 0 and full health is 1. For example, blindness may receive a QALY score of .45, male impotence a score of .8, and baldness a score of .95. Researchers can use clinical information to determine how many QALYs are gained when a patient receives a certain drug. For example, if male impotence has a QALY score of .8. then a drug that cures male impotence would create a QALY gain of .2 QALYs per year of effectiveness.

QALY scores can be used to compare the cost-effectiveness of different clinical interventions. If the cure for male impotence costs $500 and is effective for two years, then the cost per QALY gained is $1,250.[18] If the treatment for baldness costs $200 and is effective for five years, then the cost per QALY gained is $800.[19] The implication is that the baldness treatment is more cost-effective than the impotence cure. Some researchers have created "league tables" that rank drugs and other medical interventions from lowest to highest cost per QALY gained. A pharmacoeconomist might justify the expense of a drug like Viagra by showing that it ranks higher on the league table (i.e., it has a lower cost per QALY) than other drugs already on the formulary. A Canadian study suggests that treatments offering costs per QALY of less than $20,000 (in 1991 dollars) are cost-effective and should be adopted.[20]

The QALY approach is an academically based effort to rationalize the trade-off between quality and cost. It provides pharmaceutical companies with the opportunity to demonstrate to cost-conscious MCOs that some medical breakthroughs are worth the price. It remains to be seen whether MCOs, their enrollees, and the medical profession will accept such a rational approach to assessing the cost-quality trade-off.

HEALTH INFORMATION TECHNOLOGIES

Providers have instituted a host of business strategies to survive in the modern health economy. The success of all these strategies is predicated on the availability of appropriate data. Whether figuring out how to upcode or unbundle, providers need information on costs and revenues. When developing league tables, practice guidelines, or disease management programs, they need information on costs, utilization, and outcomes. Without such data, providers cannot develop their strategies, accurately predict their effects, or measure how well they have done.

In a market economy, where there is a need, there is usually a market to meet it. The need for health care data, as well as the market that has emerged to fill that need, is no exception. J. D. Kleinke, chairman of the Health Strategies Network, reports that, in 1997, the health information technologies (HIT) industry sold $15 billion worth of products to health care organizations.[21] By the year 2000, that figure is expected to reach $25 billion. The variety of HIT products is staggering: "optimization" software helps hospitals upcode; cost-accounting software helps hospitals measure their costs; outcomes software helps hospitals and other providers evaluate their quality. The growth of these HIT markets, especially in cost-accounting and outcomes measurement, is encouraging. New HIT products will make it possible for providers to better assess costs and benefits and thereby move off the flat of the curve. Unfortunately, the current HIT products are not up to the tasks at hand. The full benefits of an incentives-driven health economy cannot be achieved until HIT improves.

Measuring Costs

Even with state-of-the-art cost-accounting software, hospitals and other providers cannot accurately measure their costs, and the resulting confusion has had profound consequences for the health economy. Everything from the proliferation of outpatient facilities to the prevalence of "drive-through deliveries" is predicated on guesses about costs that could well be wrong.

The problem is best explained by means of an example. Consider estimating the cost of keeping a maternity patient in the hospital for an extra day after she has given birth. To estimate such costs, hospitals rely on accounting data, usually "legacy" accounting systems that were developed years ago to generate claims for indemnity insurers, Medicare, and Medicaid. Years ago, these payers reimbursed for costs, and legacy accounting systems report costs for each of the hospital's many "cost centers"—departments such as nursing wards, laboratories, and the laundry service. To determine the total cost of keeping a patient an extra day, the hospital adds up the additional costs that would accrue in each cost center. This sounds simple enough, but it is fraught with difficulties. To understand why, it is necessary to discuss the excruciatingly boring subject of hospital cost accounting.

Hospitals typically divide costs into direct and indirect costs. *Direct costs* are directly tied to patient care, such as nursing costs and costs of medications. It is fairly straightforward for the hospital to identify direct costs incurred when the new mother stays an extra day. *Indirect costs*, including the costs of management, information systems, and the physical plant, are not easily linked to specific patients. The new mother incurs few indirect costs when she stays an extra day, and the hospital would be hard-pressed to identify them. To determine the total cost of an extra maternity day, the hospital computes the direct cost and adds to this an "appropriate" amount of indirect costs.

Because indirect costs account for half of total costs, hospital managers understand the need for accurate indirect cost allocation. To improve accuracy, many hospitals have invested several hundred thousand dollars or more for accounting systems such as TSI, SMS, and Meditech. These systems offer a vast improvement over older cost allocation methods, which were usually chosen to maximize cost-based reimbursement rather than to measure the actual costs of care. But they are still not very accurate. One problem is that there is a lot of guesswork involved in allocating indirect costs. By definition, it is difficult to assign indirect costs to specific patients. This problem will not go away until hospitals do a better job of directly tying costs to patients—that is, until indirect costs represent a much smaller percentage of total costs.

Most hospital managers recognize how difficult it is to accurately assign indirect costs, but they may not recognize that it is also difficult to accurately assign direct costs, especially nursing costs. Different patients have different nursing needs, even when they are in the same ward. Yet existing accounting systems allocate the daily costs of nursing care equally to all patients in the ward. This can lead to gross errors in cost estimation. The relatively healthy maternity patient who stays in the hospital an extra day requires much less attention than the roommate who has just undergone a difficult delivery. Even so, hospitals usually assign the same daily nursing costs to both patients. As a result, the hospital greatly overestimates the cost of keeping the healthy new mother for the extra day.

Because of these and other errors in cost allocation, hospitals systematically overestimate certain costs and underestimate others. This is no small matter. In an incentive-driven system, the organization of health care delivery depends critically on how well providers estimate costs. Consider the conventional wisdom that it is expensive to keep postpartum maternity patients and healthy newborns in the hospital, which has led MCOs to encourage "drive-through deliveries." But once the mother and child are well enough to consider going home, their medical needs are minimal. Even if they remain in the hospital, they will typically require little more than inexpensive "hotel services" (food, clean sheets, and, for the baby, a few clean diapers). It might cost only a few dollars more to keep them in the hospital an extra day than to send them home.

Why, then, do MCOs encourage early discharges? They do it to save money. Because hospital accounting is inadequate, hospital prices are out of line with costs. Hospitals charge a lot for an extra maternity day, even if the cost is minimal, and MCOs respond to these prices by encouraging early discharges. By the same reasoning, it follows that limitations in current accounting practice have contributed to the growth in outpatient surgery, freestanding emergency rooms and clinics, and home health care.

One solution is for providers to do a better job of measuring costs and matching prices to costs. For now, state-of-the-art accounting methods used elsewhere in business, particularly *activity-based cost accounting* (ABC), are mostly foreign to the health economy. ABC requires painstaking analysis to correctly identify direct costs and link indirect costs to specific products. Given the incentives to control total costs, providers are sure to look to ABC. But ABC is very costly, and according to Bala Balachandran, a professor of accounting at the Kellogg Graduate School of Management and one of the leading proponents of ABC, only about ten hospitals nationwide had implemented the method by 1999 (that is less than 0.2 percent of all hospitals). In the meantime, some hospitals and MCOs have recognized the divergence between accounting costs and actual costs, and have adjusted prices to better reflect reality. For example, some hospitals have lowered their prices for postsurgical days by 50 percent or more.

Even if hospitals do a better job of estimating their costs, other problems with cost measurement will remain. Physicians and other providers also rely on legacy accounting systems (based on claims data) to measure their costs. But they lack the scale necessary to purchase cost-accounting software, and therefore they can only make crude guesses as to their costs. Moreover, to evaluate drug therapies, practice guidelines, or disease stage management programs, providers will have to measure the cost of an episode of illness, not just one or two parts of the episode. But, as Kleinke reports, "The most significant management challenge posed by claims data is the fragmentation of patient information."[22] Currently, there is no way to link existing provider databases to create a complete "medical record." As a result, there is no reliable way for providers to measure costs for an episode of illness.

Gradually, a number of organizations are overcoming this problem. Insurers, such as United Healthcare and many of the Blue Cross and Blue Shield plans, are constructing "quasi" medical records from their claims data. Some employers are doing the same, often with the assistance of consulting firms such as the Sachs Group in Evanston, Illinois. If the database is large enough, the organization can perform statistical analyses that compare the costs of different treatments, as well as identify providers with costly practice patterns. Claims data usually have limited clinical information however, which makes it difficult to control for differences in patient severity and to track outcomes.

Measuring Outcomes

Outcomes HIT are statistical methods used to estimate risk-adjusted quality. These methods typically compare actual outcomes of treatment (e.g., mortality, complications during recovery, ability to perform specific tasks) with the predicted outcomes (i.e., the outcomes that would be expected based on the severity of illness). Any difference is attributed to "quality." For example, if a provider's patients have low actual mortality but high predicted mortality, the methodology will lead researchers to conclude that the provider has superior quality. As I will explain in detail in Chapter 7, there are many problems with how HIT measures and predicts outcomes. Data fragmentation remains an issue as well. If a new mother suffers complications after her discharge, her hospital may not find out unless she returns to it for treatment. Nor would researchers necessarily be able to connect data across different providers. Doing so might require some kind of national health care ID, a topic I will address in Chapter 8.

MCO COMPETITION

Thanks to managed care, providers are focused on reducing costs. MCOs have been able to extract some of the savings in the form of lower payments to providers. But do they pass them along to consumers in the form of lower premiums? Although there is no direct evidence on this one way or the other, both economic theory and indirect evidence suggest that consumers are reaping some of the benefits.

The most powerful theoretical argument is that the MCO market is reasonably competitive. In most areas of the country, employers have several MCOs to choose from and tend to view them as being essentially identical. A substantial percentage of employees will switch from one MCO to another if they can save a few dollars a month.[23] These are the ingredients for fierce competition among MCOs, because each MCO knows that small differences in price can determine success or failure. The evidence is in the relatively poor financial performance of MCOs in recent years. Oxford Health Plans had the most publicized financial problems and went bankrupt, but it was not the only MCO to struggle. Harvard Pilgrim Health Plan lost $50 million in 1998; Kaiser's northeast division lost $90 million, forcing Kaiser to leave the market; and Kaiser's northern California division, one of the oldest and most successful HMOs in the nation, also lost about $100 million in 1998. The entire sector is troubled. As recently as 1997, the MCO industry had an overall pretax profit margin of just 2 percent.

Competition among MCOs helps explain why the era of double-digit inflation in health insurance premiums is over. For several years during the mid-1990s, premiums held steady or even fell. They were probably kept artificially low as MCOs sought to attract new business by setting prices below their costs. But even as some MCOs raise premiums to recoup their losses (and cover the rising costs of prescription drugs), premium increases remain well below historical levels.

Competition has reduced costs and premiums, but it threatens the long-term viability of providers and MCOs alike. Something has to give. Unable to outdo their competition, providers and MCOs are increasingly seeking another way out. The result is a second merger-and-acquisition wave in health care. Unlike the first wave in the 1970s, when national for-profit health care systems turned around the fortunes of monopoly rural hospitals, the current wave involves all kinds of providers, as well as insurers, attempting to prosper in fiercely competitive urban markets. The next chapter describes their ongoing struggle for efficiencies and market power.

CHAPTER 6

Merger Mania

THE 1990s were a decade of unprecedented consolidation in the health economy. As recently as 1975, three-fourths of all community hospitals were independent, including the vast majority of nonprofits. Today, most hospitals belong to systems. In some metropolitan areas, virtually all hospitals have found partners. There have been so many hospital mergers that the journal *Hospitals* changed its name to *Hospitals and Health Systems*, and the U.S. Federal Trade Commission (FTC) and the Department of Justice (DOJ) were forced to issue antitrust guidelines for hospital mergers. In 1975, most physicians were in solo practice; today fewer than 25 percent remain in solo practice. As more and more physician groups obtain a measure of market power, the FTC and DOJ have issued separate guidelines for physician mergers. Payers have also consolidated. At one time the Blue Cross and Blue Shield plans were the unquestioned market share leaders in their local markets. Now, mergers among for-profit MCOs are creating rivals to the Blues, and the antitrust agencies have begun to intervene in MCO mergers.

There has also been substantial restructuring along the vertical chain. In 1975, hospitals and physicians were independent of each other and had virtually no ownership interests in nursing homes, insurance companies, or freestanding outpatient facilities. During the 1980s, many hospitals expanded beyond their core inpatient business, while many physicians sacrificed autonomy and formed partnerships with hospitals. By 1993, the American Hospital Association member survey had expanded to include questions about a variety of vertical relationships. According to the most recent survey, about half of the urban community hospitals in the United States have joined with their medical staffs to form physician-hospital organizations (PHOs), which seek to reengineer the delivery the hospital services while facilitating contracting with MCOs. In addition, many hospitals have established freestanding clinics and diagnostic facilities, some of which compete with similar facilities owned by physicians. Some hospitals (and some MCOs) have even purchased physician practices.

These mergers and expansions are a direct response to managed care. As with other strategies to cope with managed care, providers hope these approaches will reduce costs or increase reimbursements. But such strategies may not always serve the best interests of consumers. Economic theory and evidence cast doubt on the extent of cost reductions, while supporting the skeptical view that many of the current mergers are thinly veiled efforts to gain market power. If current trends continue, the health care economy may be dominated by firms that succeed through the abuse of power rather than through value creation.

THE QUEST FOR POWER

When the for-profit hospital chains emerged twenty years ago, there was really little to fear. Despite the concerns expressed by my Cornell professors and others, Hospital Corporation of America, Humana, and the other chains had little chance to exercise power. Although they each owned dozens of hospitals, their holdings were scattered across the country. Because health care markets are local, this meant that the chains rarely had more than one or two hospitals in any single market. Thus, they could not consolidate services within local markets, could not assemble local networks, and, most significantly, could not exercise market power. At that time, none of these shortcomings really mattered. Hospitals had to deal with facilities planning and cost-based reimbursement; productive efficiency and market power had little to do with their success.

The emergence of managed care changed everything. Now hospitals and other providers must successfully compete within their local markets, which is why the merger wave of the 1990s is local. Whether to cut costs, boost prices, or both, providers are partnering with erstwhile competitors in their local markets. The search for a competitive edge has made for some strange bedfellows—witness the merger in St. Louis of the secular Barnes Hospital with Jewish Hospital of St. Louis and Christian Hospitals Northeast-Northwest to form the BJC hospital system.[1] Today, every metropolitan area has its share of local systems. In Chicago, the largest is the Advocate system, with ten hospitals. But Chicago also has the University of Chicago system, the Rush system, and the Evanston Northwestern system, to name just a few. Few hospitals in Chicago remain without partners. The same holds true for most other metropolitan areas.

There are so many hospitals in the Chicago market that even the Advocate system has less than a 20 percent market share. The largest systems in New York, Los Angeles, and most other big markets also have relatively small market shares, but in many smaller markets, there are systems with market shares of 30 percent or more. Restricting attention to submarkets, such as teaching hospitals or suburban hospitals, it is possible to find systems in small and large markets alike with shares exceeding 50 percent. Some physician groups are approaching similar market shares (especially within specialties). Ongoing MCO consolidation is enabling purchasers to obtain large market shares of their own.

If consolidation creates value for consumers, perhaps through cost reductions that are passed along in the form of lower prices, then all is well and good. But theory and evidence suggest that many mergers will do little more than create market power for the merging parties, allowing them to avoid the difficult decisions needed for value creation. This would deny consumers the benefits of competition and would all but spell the end to managed care.

A SPOONFUL OF THEORY

Economists use the expressions *economies of scale* and *economies of scope* to describe how costs change as firms get bigger and offer more products and services. These terms, which are often used interchangeably, may be broadened to include not only cost reductions but also quality improvements. In all cases, they mean that bigger is better. No matter what the industry, all parties to a merger can be expected to invoke the mantra of scale economies, boasting of the many "synergies" that the deal will create. Economists routinely question synergy claims, partly because economists are overly cynical, but partly because they have studied the theory and evidence. A wealth of economic research from many industries generates two basic facts about mergers: the risks are great, and the savings are usually smaller than anticipated.[2] There is no exemption for health care, where managers have found that it is a lot easier to boast about synergies than it is to realize them.

Where Do Scale Economies Come From?

There are many potential sources of scale economies. Larger firms often have a cost advantage because they can spread fixed costs across a greater volume of output.[3] Virtually all production processes, including the production of health care services, involve some fixed costs. But fixed costs do not always represent a large percentage of total costs and therefore do not always generate substantial economies of scale. Fixed costs are generally higher at firms that have invested a lot in capital equipment like buildings, machinery, and computers. Another way that large firms can enjoy lower costs is through superior inventory management, which is especially important when demand fluctuates. Larger firms can also enjoy cost savings by securing purchasing discounts from suppliers.

These potential sources of scale economies are present in health care. Hospitals have substantial fixed expenses, including the costs of high-tech services such as MRIs and neonatology wards, sterile surgical suites,

computers used for payroll and medical records keeping, and a fully
stocked pharmacy. Physicians may also incur large fixed expenses for
claims systems, medical records, and diagnostic equipment. By merging,
providers can often consolidate some of these facilities to eliminate duplicative fixed costs. For example, a hospital with two neonatology wards can
close one and shift all its neonates to the other. Providers also require staff
and equipment to handle peak loads, such as when several patients simultaneously need an MRI. William Lynk estimates that larger hospitals can
reduce expenses by 5 percent or more by efficiently managing the peak
load problem.[4]

Although there are theoretical reasons to believe that bigger is better in
medical care, this does not automatically imply that the savings from
mergers will turn out to be substantial. Fixed expenses generally account
for only a fraction of total costs. Labor accounts for 60 percent of hospital
costs and an even higher percentage of total costs for other providers such
as nursing homes, physician offices, and home health care providers. Materials may account for another 10 percent of total cost. Labor and materials costs are usually not fixed, and if two providers merge, they will not
find it easy to lay off personnel or cut back on materials unless they were
overstaffed or oversupplied prior to the merger. If that is the case, then
merging is not the only way to realize savings. Bloated providers can unilaterally cut back on staff and supplies.

Not only are the advantages of scale economies likely to be modest at
best; there may be ways for smaller providers to achieve many of these
advantages without merging. Rather than purchase costly equipment,
small providers can lease on a daily basis or enter into joint ventures with
peers to share expenses. This permits fuller utilization of the equipment
and correspondingly lower costs. Such joint ventures have become increasingly common in markets dominated by managed care. For example,
in their study of the Madison, Wisconsin, hospital market, Steven Hill and
Barbara Wolfe suggest that the growth of managed care is the sole reason
for an unprecedented number of hospital joint ventures.[5] Many providers
have joined purchasing alliances such as the Premier Health Alliance,
which has over seventeen hundred member hospitals and helps them obtain discounts on many medical supplies, including drugs and diagnostic
equipment.

There is one final strike against the scale economies rationale for mergers. Merging providers are unlikely to reap the benefits unless they integrate operations. Competing hospitals that offer duplicative open-heart
surgery or radiation oncology facilities, perhaps as a legacy of the medical
arms race, can certainly reduce costs and potentially even boost quality by
consolidating facilities under one roof. Such consolidation has been
achieved in a handful of mergers. For example, after two hospitals in Mar-

ion, Ohio, merged, all inpatient care was shifted to one, leaving the other to focus on outpatient care. But other mergers, such as the one between Stanford University Hospital and the University of California, San Francisco Medical Center did not result in substantial clinical integration and thus failed to generate substantial savings. The experience of Stanford and UCSF is typical. All too often, merging hospitals integrate one or two departments but otherwise remain operationally independent. From the perspective of achieving economies of scale, it is almost as if the hospitals never really merged. One big obstacle is that hospital medical staffs often resist operational integration, which would require all physicians at one hospital to shift their practices to an unfamiliar facility, report to a new chief of service, work with entirely new staff, and possibly even adopt a new style of practice. My colleague Mark Shanley offered an example of how physicians can block a hospital merger. He attributed the termination of merger talks between the University of Chicago Hospital and nearby Michael Reese Hospital to the failure of the hospitals' surgical staffs to agree on how to divide services and authority. Twelve years later, Michael Reese has been through two owners, including Columbia/HCA. Fred Brown, CEO of the BJC system, has faced similar obstacles in his efforts to achieve clinical integration. He describes the problem of clinical integration this way: "The real key now is to manage the cost of clinical care, and that's where the physician will continue to play a critical role. That's been our major stumbling block."[6] Physicians can even cause seemingly successful mergers to fall apart, as occurred in San Jose in the early 1990s, when fractiousness among physicians caused a local system with four member hospitals to implode.

What Do the Facts Say about Efficiencies?

Because theory is mixed on the extent to which health care mergers will generate savings, the proof must come from the data. The evidence, not surprisingly, is mixed as well. Virtually all of the research on mergers focuses on hospitals, which partly reflects the prevalence and size of hospital mergers but mainly reflects the availability of data. Studies agree that smaller hospitals have higher average costs. But there is no agreement about the magnitude of the cost differential or the size at which economies of scale are exhausted. My own research on the costs of hospital support functions (e.g., accounting, medical records, cafeteria) suggests that economies of scale are present for hospitals with up to 200 to 250 beds, with hospitals at that size enjoying a 10 to 30 percent cost advantage over smaller hospitals.[7] I find no further advantages for hospitals with more than 250 beds. Other studies "pinpoint" the size at which economies of scale are exhausted at anywhere from 100 to 1,500 beds. Many of these studies are plagued by statistical problems, and there remains little consensus on the exact nature of scale economies.[8] There have been few studies of scale economies for physician groups, largely because good cost data are not available. Given that their practices are labor-intensive, I suspect that economies of scale among physician groups are minimal.

Even if research had found consistent, unambiguous evidence of massive scale economies, this would shed little light on the benefits of mergers. Studies may show that smaller hospitals are less efficient than larger ones, but a merger between two small hospitals does not, in general, produce one large one. Unless there is operational integration, there remain two small hospitals, but with a single owner. To find out if mergers save money, it is not enough to compare hospitals of different sizes; it is necessary to study actual mergers.

Two surveys from the early 1990s provide some evidence that all was not well with mergers.[9] Administrators who had recently been through a merger generally agreed that they did not realize the anticipated savings. These survey findings were echoed in a 1999 study, published in the *McKinsey Quarterly*, which examined 300 of the 750 hospital mergers and alliances that took place between 1993 and 1998, finding "the economic advantages local hospital networks expected to derive from consolidation have largely eluded them."[10]

Systematic analysis of hospital costs by academic researchers tends to support these pessimistic findings. Mark Shanley, Amy Durkac, and I compare eleven local systems in California with independent hospitals matched for size and location. We find that they provided similar numbers of costly high-tech services and had comparable patient care costs.[11] In other words, the systems did not seem to eliminate duplicative facilities or enjoy any other cost advantage over independent hospitals.

Robert Conner and his colleagues at the University of Minnesota reach somewhat more favorable conclusions about mergers.[12] They perform a before-and-after analysis of every hospital merger in the United States between 1986 and 1994, and find, all else being equal, that the typical independent hospitals that merge reduce their costs by about 5 percent. Mergers between hospitals offering similar services generated bigger savings, supporting the idea that hospitals can save money through operational integration. Curiously, mergers in the 1980s generated greater cost reductions than did mergers in the 1990s. Perhaps the 1990s mergers were less about saving money and more about creating market power. Along these lines, mergers in concentrated markets (markets with few competitors) did not seem to generate any cost savings; perhaps they were only about market power.

A recent dissertation by Min Guo helps to reconcile these two studies.[13] Using nationwide data, Guo confirms that merged hospitals are, on average, no more efficient than independents. She also confirms that mergers do, on average, generate modest savings. Finally, she observes that the typical merging hospital is relatively inefficient prior to merging and catches up with other hospitals afterward. It seems that merging hospitals are looking for a way to become more efficient. Rather than take unilateral action, they hope that merging will solve their problems. From my experiences examining merger documents filed with the FTC, it is apparent that most merging hospitals anticipate that the largest savings will come from laying off staff. But labor costs are not fixed. If a hospital needs to lay off excess staff, it can do so without merging. Admittedly, it may be easier for managers to lay off staff as part of a merger "consolidation" than a unilateral reduction in workforce, but this is hardly a sufficient justification for merging. Perhaps the merger provides managers an excuse for layoffs.

Economies of Scale and MCOs

While the theory and evidence on efficiencies in hospital mergers are somewhat mixed, those on efficiencies in MCO mergers are less equivocal. Scale economies are small to nonexistent. MCOs are labor-intensive, with more salespeople and underwriters than bricks and mortar. There may be some scale economies associated with accumulating and analyzing claims data (e.g., to create disease management programs), but most MCOs have not made inroads in developing this expertise. We should not expect much in the way of economies of scale. In a 1996 study, Ruth Given confirms this, finding that "economies of scale provide a strong justification for mergers only in the case of relatively small HMOs."[14]

Even if they have nothing to offer by way of operational efficiencies, bigger HMOs may still have an advantage over their smaller rivals. By controlling more lives, they are usually able to obtain better prices from providers. This is the motivation behind an unwelcome trend—the effort by payers and providers alike to succeed in the health economy through the accumulation of power, rather than the creation of value.

THE OTHER MOTIVE FOR MERGERS

When it comes to justifying mergers, the managers of health care firms are no different than the managers of other firms. They say they are merging to create efficiencies, avoid duplication, and improve services; in other words, they are merging to realize synergies. More often than not, the synergies remain elusive, yet the mergers continue. Health care managers understand that even if mergers do not generate synergies, they can pay off by generating market power.

For example, in a popular merger strategy, a large tertiary care hospital acquires a smaller community hospital. This assures the former of receiving all the referrals from the latter, as well as all the profits that the referrals generate.[15] This is not a foolproof strategy. The feeder community hospital can drive up its purchase price by entertaining offers from more than one tertiary care hospital. If it is not careful, the acquirer can overpay. Moreover, once the other tertiary care hospitals in the market find they have one less referral source, they may respond by acquiring their own feeders. After this balkanization of the market, the tertiary care hospitals have about the same number of referrals as they started with, but physicians and their patients in community hospitals can no longer pick and choose their tertiary care hospital. Instead, they have little choice but to visit the acquirer. These deals have the effect of steering patients to tertiary care hospitals based on financial rather than clinical considerations.

Mergers may harm consumers in their pocketbooks as well by enabling providers to raise their prices without concomitant improvements in services. I have asked many providers why they wanted to merge. Although publicly they all invoked the synergies mantra, virtually everyone stated privately that the main reason for merging was to avoid competition and/or obtain market power. Some of managers I spoke with felt that reduced competition would benefit consumers, citing the medical arms race. But all felt threatened by MCOs and believed that by achieving some measure of market power, they could resist pressure to cut prices. On this point, both theory and evidence concur.

THE PRICE-CONCENTRATION RELATIONSHIP

The fundamental paradigm of the economics of industrial organization is that when all else is equal, prices are higher in more concentrated markets (i.e., markets with fewer competitors). This is known as the *price-concentration relationship*. There are many factors at work here, but at the heart of the price-concentration relationship is consumer shopping. As long as consumers are willing and able to shop for the best price, firms will tend to compete away their profits by reducing prices. The more firms there are, the more intense the competition.

In the traditional health economy, competition was patient-driven, and consumers did not shop around for the best price. Physicians competed through word of mouth and by getting into referral networks, not by lowering prices. Hospitals competed by attracting physicians through the medical arms race. Cost-based reimbursement rendered hospital price competition moot. Not surprisingly, researchers failed to find a price-concentration relationship at that time. If anything, prices seemed to be higher in less concentrated markets, reflecting the MAR and the higher costs of services in urban areas.

Managed care brought payer-driven competition to health care markets. Unlike their enrollees, MCOs do shop around for the best provider prices, a practice that has injected price competition into provider markets. Research on hospital pricing confirms that in markets dominated by MCOs, the traditional price-concentration relationship holds true; hospital prices are generally lower where there are more competitors.[16]

There is no direct evidence on the price-concentration relationship for other providers, largely because it is difficult to obtain the necessary price data. However, there is anecdotal evidence that physicians who face little competition can earn substantially higher than average incomes. In one antitrust case, it was revealed that the members of a monopoly radiology practice in the upper Midwest earned an average of $750,000 annually. The plaintiff in this case used the evidence of high earnings to convince the jury that the radiology group did, indeed, have a monopoly.[17]

Hospital Mergers and Antitrust

The price-concentration relationship forms the backbone of merger policy under the antitrust laws. The DOJ and FTC view mergers in concentrated markets as harmful because they generally lead to higher prices. With the advent of payer-driven competition, the DOJ and FTC have turned their attention to health care markets. They have required hundreds of merging providers to produce detailed documents justifying their deals and have sought injunctions to block over a dozen hospital mergers. Responding to the concerns of health care providers who were unsure how to act when under the antitrust microscope, they published guidelines for hospitals and physicians. These guidelines specify the types of deals the DOJ and FTC would likely try to block and also the types of deals that fall within antitrust "safety zones" and would not be challenged.

The DOJ and FTC cannot unilaterally block mergers. When they believe that a merger might be anticompetitive, they seek an injunction from a federal judge to block the deal.[18] While the antitrust agencies have successfully blocked a few mergers, judges have not always been receptive to DOJ and FTC complaints. Between 1990 and 1997, federal judges declined to block hospital mergers in small to medium-sized towns in Virginia, California, Iowa, Missouri, and Michigan. Owing to their lack of success in these cases, the DOJ and FTC have all but abandoned efforts to block mergers in larger markets, where there are nominally more competitors. These antitrust enforcement failures should trouble advocates of managed care. Selective contracting enables MCOs to obtain lower prices and change the way that providers deliver care. But hospitals with market power can resist MCO demands for change; if the hospitals have no serious competition, where else can the MCOs turn?

In virtually all of the merger cases challenged by the agencies, the merging hospitals had over 50 percent market shares in their local communities. Although these mergers seem to be anticompetitive, the courts have accepted a number of arguments to permit them. In a merger case in Roanoke, Virginia, the judge ruled that outpatient services provide ample competition to inpatient services. The judge in a Davenport, Iowa, merger case held that hospitals located in other communities (often fifty miles or more away) provide sufficient competition to prevent the merged hospitals from exploiting their market power. The judge ruling on a merger in Joplin, Missouri, threw out an FTC complaint by arguing, in effect, that the federal government had no right to meddle in local matters. After an appeals court ordered the judge to hear the case, he ruled against the FTC anyway, claiming that if patients did not like the resulting high prices, they could get care by traveling up to seventy-five miles (one way) to obtain slightly lower prices.

Many hospital mergers involve nonprofits, and many hospital managers want to use their nonprofit status as a shield against antitrust enforcement. The judge ruling on a merger between the two largest hospitals (both nonprofits) in Grand Rapids, Michigan, accepted the hospitals' claims that nonprofits are unlikely to take actions that would be costly to their communities. It would be a mistake to permit nonprofits to escape the rigors of competition. For one thing, it is getting harder to identify the nonprofits without a scorecard. Some nonprofits are operated with management eyes focused on the bottom line. Some nonprofits have complicated ownership structures involving for-profit subsidiaries, which permits them to achieve substantial profit margins in some lines of business while maintaining favorable tax status in others. But even if nonprofits remain true to their eleemosynary purposes, even if they do not raise prices as high as for-profits, and even if they sacrifice some profit to boost quality and provide uncompensated care, we should not turn a blind eye to nonprofit mergers. There is no substitute for competition to motivate the quest for efficiency and innovation. Perhaps we are better off with nonprofit hospitals than with for-profits (though the jury is out on this one), but we are definitely better off with competing nonprofits than with monopoly nonprofits.

These antitrust cases may seem to be of limited importance, since only a small fraction of Americans live in communities with three or four hospitals. But as hospitals (and other providers) continue to consolidate, a handful of systems are coming to dominate even large metropolitan areas, including Boston, Minneapolis, and Cleveland. Two or three systems may not be enough to assure competition, and any further consolidation would all but end any pretense of it.

Even if systems do not dominate entire metropolitan areas, consolidation in submarkets can limit competition. Hospitals in neighboring suburban communities are merging. So, too, are teaching hospitals in larger metropolitan areas. As a result, MCOs find it increasingly difficult to assemble viable networks without dealing with the merged hospitals. In 1997, the DOJ unsuccessfully challenged a merger between two teaching hospitals on Long Island. The court's ruling in favor of the merger essentially forces MCOs to either contract with the merged hospitals or send their enrollees to tertiary care hospitals in New York City. It remains to be seen whether Long Island residents will be paying more for tertiary care services as a result. This merger is just the tip of the iceberg. The 1997 merger between Stanford University Hospital and the University of California, San Francisco Medical Center, created a tertiary care juggernaut that could have tremendous clout with purchasers, if it survives long enough to overcome resistance to integration and cutbacks in Medicare payments to teaching hospitals. Look for even more consolidation in the future as hospitals seek to avoid the ravages of competition.

Doctor Welby Joins the Fray

It is not so easy for physicians to obtain market power. A town with three hospitals may have a dozen cardiologists, twenty radiologists, and even more PCPs. Many of these physicians will belong to groups, but in most metropolitan areas the groups have relatively tiny market shares. Despite the abundant competition, physicians, especially PCPs, do have some power. Physicians often recommend specific MCOs to their patients, and many consumers select their MCO on the basis of whether their physician is in the network. But many physicians are unwilling to test their power by holding out for higher prices. One reason is that MCOs will occasionally play hardball with physicians; the MCOs will exclude some high-price PCPs from their provider networks even if they end up losing some enrollees. A more subtle reason is that most physicians are loyal to their patients and will stay in MCO networks to assure continuity of care, even if this means they must offer deep discounts.

The MCOs seem to be slightly ahead in the power struggle, at least as evidenced by slight declines in physician incomes brought about by managed care. Seeking to regain their footing, some physicians have engaged in practices that have caught the attention of the DOJ and FTC. In the most blatant examples of questionable activities, independent physicians have formed organizations whose sole purpose, apparently, is to negotiate contracts with MCOs. While this is not illegal per se, the physicians sometimes set prices collectively and agree not to sign MCO contracts except as part of the organization. This blatant price-fixing violates antitrust laws. Antitrust agencies have challenged several of these efforts, forcing the dissolution of a large physician group in Phoenix and forcing a physician group in Mesa, Colorado, to sign a consent decree pertaining to price-fixing. The antitrust agencies have also challenged collective bargaining arrangements in Michigan (the entire Michigan State Medical Society was involved) and Tuscon, Arizona (in a criminal action involving dentists). These few cases have sent a chill down the spine of physicians seeking a way to gain the upper hand on MCOs.

Physicians are slowly learning the dos and don'ts of antitrust law. They know that if they belong to a group, they may collectively set prices. In some places, however, physician groups are so large that they may constitute monopolies. Dominant groups in Dallas–Ft. Worth, Texas; Sioux Falls, South Dakota; Billings, Montana; and Park Ridge, Illinois, have all been placed under the antitrust microscope either by the federal antitrust agencies or by private parties who feel they have been harmed by antitrust abuses. Physicians who belong to a physician practice management firm may also set prices collectively. There is some concern that eventually PPMs may own enough physician practices to achieve market power, though the recent collapse of MedPartners has alleviated this fear.

Many physicians who would like to regain some control over their pricing do not want to give up their autonomy to PPMs or partner into giant groups. Physician advocacy groups such as the American Medical Association have backed legislation that would enable physicians to coordinate prices while otherwise remaining independent. The AMA has even embraced unionization. I will return to these topics in Chapter 8.

MCO MERGERS

MCOs are steadfastly opposed to any and all activities that would enhance provider market power. They have testified in support of DOJ and FTC efforts to block mergers. They have also lobbied against legislation that would exempt providers from antitrust scrutiny. This comes as no surprise. If providers obtain market power, they can hold out for higher prices, resist the implementation of UR, and otherwise thwart managed care strategies. When that happens, MCOs look exactly like indemnity insurers and lose their raison d'être.

Providers counter that MCOs have all the power and that they need to level the playing field. This is a bit simplistic. It is true that even the smallest MCOs have a certain degree of power relative to individual providers, but only because they are willing to shop around for the best price. This is no different from the power enjoyed by consumers in all competitive markets, such as when home buyers shop around for the best mortgage rate. There is nothing wrong with consumer power; it is the engine that drives competitive markets toward efficiency.

MCOs have realized that consumer power alone does not guarantee profitability, however. The reason has to do with a fundamental tenet of business strategy: no matter how efficient a firm may be, it cannot make a profit unless it is differentiated from its competitors or it enjoys lower costs. Differentiation appears to be difficult. Most MCOs go about the business of shopping for medical care in the same way, using nearly identical provider networks, similar payment rules, and the same handful of UR agencies. There may be differences in how they pay providers or enforce access restrictions, but these are subtle and difficult for consumers to detect. In the eyes of employers and employees shopping around for an MCO, most MCOs seem pretty much alike. Because MCOs are largely undifferentiated, the resulting competition has been brutal, and profit margins have been thin.

If an MCO cannot differentiate itself from its rivals, the only way for it to survive is by reducing costs. The best way to do this is to reduce what it pays to providers, and the best way to do this is to increase its purchasing clout. Two of the largest payers, Medicare and Blue Cross, have been doing this for years. By virtue of their size, Medicare and Blue Cross have not had to shop around for the best prices. Instead, they name their price and their payment method. Medicare imposed its PPS on hospitals and the RBRVS on physicians. Many Blue Cross plans not only demand and get steep discounts but also force providers to accept "most favored nation" clauses that guarantee that Blue Cross pays the lowest price of any payer.[19] (These clauses are not always bad for providers because they can limit the incentives of providers to cut prices for other insurers.[20]) Most providers are so dependent on Medicare and Blue Cross that they have little choice but to accept these terms or risk bankruptcy. By way of contrast, most providers are not as dependent on Medicaid, and some have refused to take Medicaid patients when payments fall too low.

MCOs learned a valuable lesson from the Blues, Medicare, and Medicaid: size matters. Many MCOs believe that the only certain way to survive is to get bigger discounts, and this means having the most covered lives. The result is an MCO merger wave, including Aetna's acquisition of NYL-Care and its recently approved merger with Prudential. The combined Aetna-Prudential MCO will control over 22 million covered lives. Another megamerger between United Healthcare and Humana fell apart in late 1998 amid gigantic second-quarter losses for United. Even so, it seems likely that MCOs will continue to consolidate. Indeed, in March 2000, Wellpoint offered to acquire Aetna to create the largest MCO in the nation. This would permit Wellpoint to assemble the data necessary to advance the practice of disease management, one of the stated goals of the merger. It should be possible to combine data without an outright merger, for example, through a joint venture dedicated to disease management. But the merger would surely increase Wellpoint/Aetna's purchasing clout.

But Is This a Good Thing?

Giant MCOs can command lower prices from providers. But is this necessarily good for consumers? The Department of Justice apparently thinks not. Concerned that the combined Aetna-Prudential MCO would control too many lives, the DOJ sought and obtained a consent decree whereby Aetna divested its interests in Dallas and Houston, two markets where both Aetna and Prudential had large market shares prior to the merger. One DOJ concern is that if MCOs get too big, they will not have to pass cost savings along to employers and employees. I am not too concerned about this threat, however. As the Twin Cities experience shows, many employers are willing to bypass MCOs if necessary to secure the benefits of lower prices for themselves.

A more disturbing possibility is that powerful MCOs—or powerful employer groups, for that matter—will reduce payments by so much that providers will respond by cutting quality. We have seen providers do this in response to Medicaid cutbacks, and the underlying theory is identical. Individual MCOs may not worry much about the quality effect, in part because they can free ride off the more generous payments of their competitors. Remember that providers often adopt a similar practice style for all their patients. Providers who receive low payments from a powerful MCO may still offer high quality if they have enough high-paying patients in other MCOs. But as MCOs consolidate further, each of the handful of MCOs will be able to extract substantial price concessions. Faced with declining payments, providers would have to reduce services to all patients. This is not necessarily a bad thing. To the extent we are still on or near the flat of the curve, some limited reductions in services may be called for. But deep reductions in services, with concomitant reductions in quality, may not be worth the savings.

In the long run, reductions in MCO payments may also drive providers from the market. This happened in the 1960s and 1970s, when reductions in Medicaid hospital payments forced many rural and inner-city hospitals to close, and it may be happening now to physicians. Just as surging demand drove up the nation's supply of physicians in the 1960s, declining demand is slowly drying up the supply. Applications to medical school declined by 17 percent between 1996 and 1999, and physicians are migrating away from states with high MCO penetration.[21] While it is possible to argue that prices can be too low, there is no way to know what the "right" MCO price is. With the complex combination of incentive problems in the market, it is impossible to determine whether we have too many or too few physicians, or receive too many or too few services.

Market Power and Value Creation

Debates about MCO market power that focus on how much MCOs pay to physicians miss a more important point. The great virtue of managed care is its potential to force providers and payers to create value, through either lower costs or higher quality. Value creation has been a hallmark of the American experiment with managed care (witness innovations such as capitation, networks, treatment guidelines, disease management, utilization review, physician practice management, pharmacoeconomics, and cost accounting). While the jury is out regarding the ultimate value of these innovations, there would be much less impetus to advance on these and other frontiers without managed care. The great danger from mergers is that they permit providers and MCOs to prosper without creating value for consumers.

Unfortunately, the courts have been less than stalwart in preserving competition in health care. It seems likely that the courts will tolerate mergers as long as there are two or more competitors in each market, and they will sometimes tolerate mergers that create local monopolies. Interestingly, the courts are more likely to block mergers when local employers and community members speak out against them. But many employers and community activists vocally support local mergers. Moreover, many people still buy into the notion that competition drives up health care costs, and they fail to understand the paradigm shift that accompanied the rise of payer-driven competition. Until the public protests, providers and purchasers will continue to ride the merger wave. The spoils of the health economy will go not to the organizations that create the most value but to those with the most power.

VERTICAL INTEGRATION

Vertical integration, which places two or more types of organizations under common ownership, is widespread throughout the health economy, as evidenced by the ongoing acquisition of physician practices by hospitals and MCOs, the establishment of physician-owned diagnostic testing facilities, and physician-hospital organizations.[22] Integrated delivery systems (IDSs) are the zenith of vertical integration. IDSs such as the Henry Ford Clinic in Michigan and Allina Healthcare in the Twin Cities place hospitals, doctors, insurance, diagnostic testing, home health care, and so forth, under a single organizational umbrella. Vertical integration usually does not pose an antitrust risk, nor does it offer obvious benefits in terms of economies of scale. Vertical integration occurs for a variety of subtle reasons. It is difficult to understand and difficult to make successful.

Vertical integration makes sense if joining organizations under common ownership enables them to create value that they could not create independently. This sounds easy, but there are many wrong reasons to integrate. Firms often vertically integrate as a way of entering a profitable business, but this is no guarantee of profitability. Many doctors opened outpatient surgical facilities after witnessing hospitals prospering in this market. But most doctors have been unable to match the scale and scope economies enjoyed by hospitals. When MCOs inject price competition into the market, the high-cost doctor-owned facilities run into trouble.

Another shaky justification for vertical integration is to tie up distribution channels. Merck, Lilly, and SmithKline bought PBMs in part to assure the sales of their own drugs. But these deals have not created value for consumers, many of whom speculated that the drug maker–controlled PBMs were no longer impartial and preferred to deal with independent PBMs. Besides, the PBMs did not come cheap. It cost Lilly $4 billion to purchase PCS, and Smith-Kline Beecham $2.3 billion to purchase DPS. Their failures to create value were costly. Lilly ended up selling PCS to Rite Aid for $1.5 billion, and SmithKline sold DPS to Express Scripts (another PBM) for $700 million.

Hospitals have tried to tie up distribution channels as well, by purchasing M.D. practices. The economic logic is identical to the one motivating tertiary care hospital acquisitions of community hospitals—to increase profitable referrals. This strategy destroys value for consumers, who lose freedom of choice, but it can be profitable for the hospital and physicians, at least in the short run. But many hospital managers with whom I have spoken have grown disillusioned with the strategy. They claim that once they acquire physician practices, their employee-physicians no longer work as hard as they did when they were independent. At the same time, independent doctors begin gravitating toward rival hospitals. Ultimately, the market is balkanized, with doctors receiving substantial sums to align themselves with individual hospitals. The hospitals are collectively worse off because they have to pay physicians for admissions (through the payment for the practice) that they used to receive for free. Patients are worse off because their physicians no longer can freely choose the hospital. But physicians come out all right, at least in their bank accounts.

Good Reasons to Integrate

Ultimately, value creation comes down to the decisions made by individuals—decisions regarding how hard to work, how much to invest in their relationships with others, which new ideas to pursue and which to disregard, and how much to sacrifice for the greater good. The market generally forces individuals to be efficient and innovative, but the market mechanisms that govern individual decision making—contracts, reputations, repeat purchases, and word of mouth—do not always work. We have seen, for example, that health care providers can persistently make the wrong treatment recommendations and yet still retain their patient and referral bases. Sometimes the market allows individuals and firms to act inefficiently or selfishly without repercussions.

Individuals within integrated firms are governed by internal control mechanisms. If they fail to be efficient and innovative, their coworkers may shun them, they may fail to obtain higher pay and greater prestige, and they can even be fired. In this way, integration replaces the hard-edged but uncertain discipline of the market with the discipline provided by corporate culture, politics, and governance. This enables the integrated firm to create value in several ways. First, integration helps protect investments that individuals make in each other. For example, a hospital-based home nursing team can invest time and effort in learning treatment protocols for ventilator dependent patients, knowing that the hospital CEO is unlikely to renege on commitments to compensate them for their efforts. Though this is an important reason for integration in many industries, health care organizations considering integration often overlook such protection of investments. Integration also facilitates data development and use. For example, providers in an IDS could adopt uniform health care information systems and share the clinical information needed to develop disease management programs. This was cited as a major justification for a proposed joint venture between physicians and a suburban Chicago hospital to open a specialized heart hospital. But some integrated providers, such as Kaiser-Permanente, have done little to exploit opportunities for generating and using integrated data systems.

The most common justification for integration is not to protect investments or to unify data systems. Rather, it is to get different providers to "eat out of the same pie." But successful implementation of the pie theory of integration has proven elusive.

The Pie Theory of Integration

In the 1980s, those bent on cost containment invoked what I call the "pie theory" of integration. According to this theory, the health care budget is the pie. Providers order services, which represent "bites" out of the pie. The ultimate goal is to leave a little pie left over. The theory has it that independent providers have no reason to share and therefore take large bites; providers will take smaller bites if they share the same goal, that is, if they realize that they are all "eating out of the same pie."

I first heard versions of this theory after the implementation of Medicare's PPS. Medicare's DRG-based payment represented the pie. Each hospital service ordered by physicians represented a bite out of the pie. For the hospital and its medical staff to survive—for there to be any pie left over—they would all have to take smaller bites. The theory sounded attractive as a motivational device, but it failed as an incentive device. Physicians continued to receive fee-for-service payments from HCFA, so no matter how much the hospital CEO urged them to take little bites, they continued to act as if they were at an all-you-can eat M.D. buffet. It is here that supporters of integration made the following logical leap: if managers want physicians to realize they are sharing the pie, it is necessary to join them together with the hospital in the same organization. That is, it is necessary for providers to vertically integrate.

The most extreme example of pie theory–driven integration is the IDS. These systems offer the entire gamut of health care services under the same corporate umbrella. Supporters claim that with everyone in the system sharing the pie, the IDS is sure to be efficient. Economist James Robinson invokes the pie theory this way: "The potential advantages of integrated delivery systems . . . are obvious. Cooperation between physicians and hospitals can encourage efficient use of services."[23] Robinson is quick to point out, however, that "some of the advantage of cooperation between physicians and hospitals can be achieved through contractual means." In other words, integration per se is not the key to preserving the pie. Rather, success or failure depends on whether the discipline and incentives provided within the integrated organization are superior to the discipline and incentives of the market.

There are few incentives within an IDS that cannot be duplicated by the market. For example, insurers can capitate independent providers just as easily as IDSs can provide fixed budgets to internal divisions. But organizational discipline can accomplish some things that the market cannot. An IDS can adopt uniform data entry and collection technology. It can use these data to develop disease management programs and use the authority of a central office to impose the program on all its members. It can encourage medical teams to invest the time required to develop specialized programs in cancer care, treatment of ventilator-dependent patients, AIDS care, and so forth, and use bonuses and promotions to reward those members who give up their time on behalf of the organization.

Although theory suggests that the IDS can accomplish many things that the free market cannot, there is no evidence of these accomplishments. Most significantly, IDSs have not met the market test. Once touted as the future of the health economy, they are enjoying decidedly mixed success as business models. Some are growing, some have failed, and many are shrinking their boundaries by spinning off services. Kaiser plans—the largest IDSs—have fared particularly poorly, with plans in New England and northern California each losing nearly $100 million in 1998. This mixed track record casts doubt on the pie theory of integration, a view that is reinforced by the lackluster performance of physician-hospital organizations.

Physician-Hospital Organizations

Physician-hospital organizations (PHOs) are an outgrowth of the pie theory. I initially heard about PHOs in the late 1980s, at a meeting of leading Illinois hospital executives. In fact, I first heard the pie theory when the CEO of one of the first hospitals in the state to offer a PHO actually stated that the PHO would force physicians and the hospital to realize that they were eating out of the same pie. Originally, PHOs were organized in response to Medicare's PPS. They derived most of their revenue from the PPS hospital reimbursements and compensated physicians partly on the basis of PHO financial performance. Hence, if the Medicare PPS payments exceeded hospital costs, the hospital would reward the PHO. By the end of the 1980s, about 10 percent of urban hospitals had PHOs. The PHOs eventually proved to be an attractive conduit for contracting with MCOs. Today, nearly half of all urban hospitals have PHOs, and many MCOs contract directly with these organizations to provide all physician and hospital services in exchange for a single capitated fee. Most PHOs share a similar organizational structure: most are for-profit; the hospital owns the PHO, either wholly or in partnership with some physicians; and all members of the medical staff are invited to participate in the PHO, though not all on an ownership basis.

Despite the intuitive appeal of the pie theory, most PHOs are struggling to hold down costs, and many suffer from bitter divisions among PCPs, specialists, and the hospital. The problem with applying the pie theory to PHOs is that individual providers, not big organizations, make medical decisions. If independent providers drive up costs to enrich themselves, so, too, will integrated providers, unless integration changes their incentives. But organizers of PHOs have often failed to make sufficient changes to incentives. PHOs usually capitate their PCPs for their services. This has the beneficial effect of encouraging the PCPs to keep their patients healthy but the perverse effect of encouraging PCPs to refer their patients to higher cost specialists. Most specialists who participate in PHOs (either as members or at the receiving end of referrals) continue to receive fee-for-service payment and have little reason to change their behavior.

PHOs are now attempting to rein in specialist expenses by increasing capitation payments to PCPs while deducting for the costs of their referrals to specialists. Thus, PCPs take a financial hit every time they refer out a patient who needs a lot of medical attention. There is a risk that PCPs will limit their referrals, which could translate into poorer outcomes. But there is also the possibility that PCPs will try to refer patients to the most cost-effective specialists. To help PCPs develop more economical referral patterns, PHOs must provide them with information about specialist practice styles. Until recently, this information has been lacking, but a few PHOs are developing the necessary information systems and instructing their members in how to use them. The changes can be dramatic. A PHO administrator told me about a PCP who lost nearly 20 percent of his income to high referral costs. After intensive data analysis, the PHO discovered that this was entirely due to referrals to one particularly costly chiropractor. Apparently, the chiropractor scheduled five times as many office visits for his patients as was normal. The PHO now provides this information to its PCPs and specialists, and referral costs are falling. (The costly chiropractor lost his referrals.)

It is difficult to generalize about PHOs from a few case studies. I tell my students that if they can imagine an incentive scheme, then some organization has tried it. For example, some PHOs capitate their specialists by paying them a fixed fee for each patient who selects the PHO to be his or her caregiver. Of course, this gives the specialists incentives to undertreat patients. Some PHOs limit incentives for undertreatment by increasing the capitated fee for physicians whose patients require extra care. But unless this adjustment perfectly accounts for medical need (as opposed to treatments rendered), it reinstates the incentives to provide excessive utilization.

Finding the Right Incentives

Imagine that incentives can be ranked on a scale from 1 to 10, where 1 is capitation, 10 is fee-for-service, and capitation adjusted for medical need is something in between. MCOs, IDSs, and PHOs devote much of time and energy to finding the "right" number along this continuum. This effort is doomed to fail, however, because it attempts to realize several goals—efficiency in production, appropriate utilization, appropriate referrals, and high quality—with a single instrument. To create maximum value, health care organizations must combine innovative incentives with information. This requires data systems that profile provider practice patterns and patient outcomes and, in some cases, track the entire medical care process. But the data systems are costly (upward of $2 million for a system to serve a physician group and even more for a system for an IDS) and are much better at evaluating cost than quality.

Of course, the most common complaint about managed care is that market forces put too much emphasis on cost at the expense of quality. But the market can be a force for high quality, not just low prices. Whether the modern health economy is able to combine the best of both is the topic of the next chapter.

CHAPTER 7

Quality

HEALTH CARE QUALITY is a slippery concept, both subjective and multidimensional. Yet patients, providers, and payers talk about it all the time; if it were not for concerns about quality, there would be no debate about the merits of managed care. To sensibly discuss quality, we need a sensible definition. For the sake of defining quality, consider the following choices: Would a patient with a major illness prefer a dispassionate doctor whose exceptional skills lead to a complete recovery or a warmly sympathetic doctor whose mediocrity leaves the patient a cripple or worse? Would an asymptomatic patient prefer a curt, clinical doctor whose knowledge of preventive medicine leads to the ordering of a lifesaving diagnostic test or a chatty, personable doctor who fails to order that test but eventually provides comfort to the dying patient's family? These are straw-men comparisons for sure, but they serve to demonstrate that while compassion and communication are important to patients, surely what matters most is the doctor's ability to prevent and cure illness. One reason that compassion and communication are so important is that they can be helpful to achieving good outcomes. But outcomes usually matter most. Simply stated, good health care providers take good care of their patients' health.

While patients undoubtedly care about outcomes, they often fail to look beyond the veneer of compassion and communication when selecting their providers. But no amount of compassion and communication can undo the damage of a missed diagnosis, delayed treatment, inappropriate prescription, unsteady surgical technique, failure to address mental health as well as physical health needs, or any number of other mistakes that a provider might make. By ignoring outcomes, consumers may be making a big mistake of their own. There is evidence of substantial variation in the quality of health care providers. There is undoubtedly some variation in the quality of MCOs as well. The laws of statistics are inviolable: half of all providers are no better than average; the same applies to MCOs. Patients have much to gain or lose by their choices of providers and MCOs.

Until recently, patients have had an excuse for ignoring outcomes when selecting providers—information about outcomes was virtually nonexistent. As a result, most patients still shop for medical care the old-fashioned way. They seek out PCPs they can trust and they rely on them for referrals to specialists and hospitals. But outcomes measurement is improving. As these measures proliferate, and as patients learn how to use them, perhaps patients will be able to augment their trust with facts.

WHY PAY ATTENTION TO QUALITY?

For those who foresee a thriving health care economy based on market principles, the stakes in quality measurement are high. A fundamental tenet of market competition is that markets provide what consumers demand. Thus far, providers and insurers have gotten the message that consumers demand cost containment. Health care markets have two features that make it imperative that consumers also demand quality. First, quality varies. Noted health services research Robert Brook puts it bluntly: "Thousands of studies . . . have shown that the level of quality care provided to the average person leaves a great deal to be desired and, perhaps more importantly, the variation in quality of care by physician or by hospital is immense."[1] There may be some goods and services for which all sellers offer pretty much the same quality—personal computers, dry cleaning, and gasoline come to mind—and there is little to be gained by shopping for the best quality. Health care is not one of them. Second, high quality is important. While quality is almost always important, there are some goods and services where the difference between low and high quality really matters. Health care is one of them. Given the importance of quality, it is likely that if the market continues to emphasize cost without commensurate concern for quality, patients will surely end up getting what they pay for.

Quality Varies

Licensing and certification go a long way toward establishing a floor for provider quality. But there is substantial variation above the floor. I have already noted the tremendous variation in practice patterns; providers use markedly different strategies for treating patients with the same disease. Unless there is a large gray area of appropriate treatment, it stands to reason that outcomes will vary as well. Some patients receive surgery they do not need and are unnecessarily exposed to iatrogenic risks, while others go without needed care. Variations are not restricted to surgical interventions. Scott Stern and Manuel Trajtenberg show that some physicians tailor drug prescriptions to their patient's specific needs, but others fail to match patients to "the drug which most suits their particular conditions."[2]

Even if patients with similar conditions receive the same treatments, they may still experience different outcomes. Harold Luft, John Bunker, and Alain Enthoven's pioneering work in the 1970s shows that more experienced providers attained better surgical results for their patients.[3] More recent studies consistently show that mortality rates for a wide variety of inpatient treatments can vary across hospitals by a factor of two or more, and that experience is but one determinant of mortality.[4] The differences in mortality rates are sometimes startling. Whereas the mean mortality rate for cardiac surgery is around 3 deaths per 100 patients, patients who go to some hospitals die twice as often, at a rate of 6 per 100, while patients who go to the best hospitals die at a rate of 2 per 100 or lower. There are similar differences in hospital mortality rates for the treatment of pneumonia, heart attack, and stroke. Outcomes differences manifest themselves in more than just mortality rates. The consulting firm HCIA reports that the interquartile range (i.e., the range from the 25th to the 75th percentile) for the surgical complication rate at U.S. hospitals is 2.64 to 5.37 per 1,000 patients; for wound infection the range is 5.96 to 10.71; for reopening the surgical site the range is 0.66 to 2.26.[5]

Some of the measured variations in outcomes may be due to unmeasured differences in illness severity. But another conclusion seems inescapable: some providers are better than others. A recent study of top-ranking hospitals brings this point home. The study examines the factors underlying the success of hospitals ranked by *U.S. News and World Report* as being among the nation's best.[6] Patients with acute myocardial infarction who were treated at the "best" hospitals had significantly lower mortality rates than patients treated elsewhere. One major reason: the best hospitals were more likely to prescribe aspirin and beta-blockers. After controlling for the use of these drugs, the differences in mortality were no longer statistically significant. Thus, some hospitals do a better job of getting appropriate medications to their patients. This difference cannot be attributed to differences in illness severity.

It should come as no surprise that quality varies across providers. Quality starts with physicians. Even going into medical school, some future doctors are more capable than others. As Robert Brook reports, the brightest medical students are segregated from poorer students throughout their training, and then later on when they obtain their hospital affiliations. This segregation exacerbates quality differences among both physicians and hospitals. Other factors contribute to quality differences among physicians: some surgeons have steadier hands; physicians do not keep equally abreast of new clinical research, do not share in the same referral networks, and do not command the same technology and staff support; and physicians do not make the same effort to heal their patients. These differences manifest themselves in many ways: diagnostic accuracy, appropriateness of treatment plans, and success of implementation. The Advisory Board suggests that there may be substantial variation among physicians in the quality of many areas of clinical practice, including pain management, wound management, and infection control.[7]

It seems that patients have much to gain, maybe even their lives, by paying attention to quality rankings. But just as provider quality varies, so too does the quality of quality rankings! The same research team that examines the *U.S. News* rankings also examines the rankings reported by HCIA and William Mercer.[8] They find no mortality differences between the top-ranked hospitals and average hospitals, instead attributing the rankings to differences in other indicators of "quality" used by HCIA and Mercer, including financial and operating factors. But these indicators may have nothing to do with how well the hospitals heal their patients.

There is likely to be variation in the quality of MCOs, though it is not clear how much to expect. On the one hand, MCOs use similar provider networks and choose from the same few UR agencies. On the other hand, MCOs use slightly different capitation rules, pay slightly different fees, and have different tolerances for referrals and departures from treatment guidelines. In a variety of subtle ways, these differences can translate into meaningful quality differences.

Valuing Quality

Consumers will pay more for high-quality goods and services if they believe that the value they receive is worth the higher cost. The same logic applies to medical care. In some cases, good-quality medical care is also low-cost care, as when a physician does appropriate diagnostic screening. But in many cases quality is expensive. It is costly to improve the precision of diagnostic tests or provide twenty-four-hour nursing. The best providers (or, at least, those who are perceived to be the best) often charge more than the rest.

Is better quality medical care worth the cost? The answer seems obvious, until one considers the size of the health economy (over $1 trillion) and the other pressing social and personal needs that could be filled if we saved some money by sacrificing just a little quality. Economists say that a good or service is "worth it" if the dollar value enjoyed by the consumer exceeds the price. Good-quality medical care can make the difference between life and death, so the value of good-quality medical care is the value of life itself. But what is this value? It is not infinite. Infinite value would imply, quite absurdly, that it is worth all of society's resources just to save one life. But societal resources are scarce, and no one would seriously suggest adding 1 percent to the health care budget, let alone spending all of society's resources, to save one life.

As with all other goods and services, it is possible to draw a line between health care services that are worth the cost and those that are not. At least when it comes to "health-improving" goods and services, most individuals already make such distinctions. To take an extreme example, very few people, even those of great means, would spend an extra $50,000 to have their cars armor-plated, although that would surely reduce their risk of a traffic fatality. Consider as a more tangible example the fact that many well-informed consumers refuse to buy air bags for their cars, preferring to spend their money on other things. There are countless other examples where consumers have confronted the trade-off between health and wealth. Some consumers pay more for pesticide-free produce, thereby reducing their cancer risk by a tiny amount, but most consumers do not. Some consumers install elaborate safety and fire prevention devices in their homes, but most consumers do not. Government agencies also have to rationalize expenditures on health and safety. Some, but not all, local governments place concrete barriers between lanes on the highway; others remove lead from school playgrounds. In each instance, someone has made a judgment regarding whether the reduction in health risk is worth the cost.

Economists have extensively studied one aspect of the economy in which the trade-off between health and wealth is often explicit. In a 1975 article, Richard Thaler and Sherwin Rosen observe that firms must increase wages to get workers to take on risky jobs, and, conversely, that workers are willing to give up some wages in exchange for a safer workplace.[9] Using data on wages and job risk, they determine how much workers value improved workplace safety. Thaler and Rosen's paper precipitated many other studies using ever more detailed data. In a review of this literature, W. Kip Viscusi concludes that workers would be willing to give up approximately $4,000 to $8,000 in wages to reduce the risk of job-site mortality by 0.1 percent.[10] (Put another way, employers have to pay workers $4,000 to $8,000 extra to take a job with an elevated mortality risk of 0.1 percent.) This works out to $4 to $8 million per life. In other words, a large group of workers must be paid an aggregate of $4 to 8 million in extra wages to take on a risk that will, in likelihood, cause one worker to die. In a subsequent review of research using similar methods, George Tolley, Donald Kenkel, and Robert Fabian report a figure of $75,000 to $175,000 per year of life saved.[11]

These values represent economists' best estimates of the value of a life (or the value of a year of life). They are based on actual choices made by individuals facing real risks to life and limb. Lest one think that only economists would have the audacity to perform such a computation, note that there are many other contexts in which someone places a dollar value on life. Juries in wrongful death suits must determine how much to award the deceased's estate. The National Institutes of Health (NIH) use "value of life" studies to determine the benefits of clinical research. Both juries and the NIH give substantial weight to the lost earnings potential of the deceased and usually report a value of life that is much smaller than the economists' figure.

Though coldly rational, the economic approach places hard numbers on something patients already know—if good-quality medical care increases the chances of living, it is worth almost any price. If anything, the economic approach serves to highlight just how much patients would be willing to pay for good health. Tests and procedures that seem expensive may actually be great bargains. Suppose that the value of a year of life is $100,000. Then a diagnostic test that increases the chances of surviving an additional ten years by just 0.1 percent is worth $1,000. A drug that increases the chances of surviving another five years by just .005 percent (one chance in 20,000) is worth $250. A $50,000 heart transplant need only extend the recipient's life by six months to justify the expense. By this assessment, new technologies that seem expensive may actually be bargains. In a recent study, David Cutler and Elizabeth Richardson examine new (since 1960) technologies for the treatment of a range of conditions, including arthritis, diabetes, and heart disease.[12] Using economic estimates of the value of a life, they conclude that even though new technologies are often very expensive, their overall benefit-to-cost ratio is about 3 to 1.

Given that life is valuable, it stands to reason that there is much to be gained by identifying the best providers. If heart transplant patients survive ten years, it is worth $20,000 to steer patients to heart surgeons whose mortality rates are 2 percent less than average. One can debate whether patients should have to bear this expense themselves or whether it should be shared by all of society. But no matter who ultimately bears the expense, the information that allows patients to identify and utilize the best quality providers is likely to be a tremendous bargain.

Using QALYs to Allocate Health Resources

Most medical interventions do not save lives, but they may improve the quality of life. Many medical researchers who are reluctant to embrace the economic approach to valuation have welcomed a methodology for comparing the relative benefits of different treatments. The methodology, based on the Quality Adjusted Life Year (QALY) scale described in Chapter 5, does not assess whether a given treatment is worth the cost but does assess whether it is more worthwhile than another treatment. By avoiding the thorny problem of placing a dollar value on life, it paves the way for broader acceptance of using cost-effectiveness criteria in medical decision making.

Recall how QALYs work.[13] A year of full health is worth 1 QALY, and a "year of death" is worth 0 QALYs. Ten years of full health are worth 10

QALYs, and so forth. All other health states (e.g., blindness, needing assistance with walking, incontinence) receive a score between 0 and 1. QALY researchers use a variety of survey methods to score health states based on how individuals value them. Survey questions include asking respondents to place health states along the scale and asking respondents how many years of life they would give up to avoid having to live with less than full health. (If the respondent would give up many years of life to avoid a particular health state, then that health state must be very undesirable.)

Once the QALY scale is developed, it is relatively straightforward to compute the cost per QALY gained from a particular medical intervention. Chapter 5 offered an example comparing the costs per QALY for treating baldness and male impotence. Here is another example. Suppose that blindness scores .45 on the QALY scale, suggesting that blindness is not quite half as "good" as full health. Curing an otherwise healthy individual's blindness for one year generates a QALY improvement of .55. Curing blindness for ten years generates a QALY improvement of 5.5. If the treatment costs $110,000 and is effective for ten years, then the cost per QALY gained is $110,000/5.5 = $20,000.

Purchasers can compare the estimated cost per QALY for the blindness treatment with estimates for other interventions to determine which ones they should pay for. It turns out that $20,000 per QALY is not exceptionally high. There are many common medical interventions, such as multiple-vessel coronary artery bypass surgery and dialysis for end-stage renal disease, that have higher costs per QALY. If purchasers are willing to pay for the latter treatments, they should also be willing to pay for the blindness treatment, which provides more QALY "bang" for the health care buck.

Although there are many unresolved issues with the QALY methodology, including how to combine survey results, how to deal with chronic conditions, and how to treat lifetime costs of disease, it has two highly attractive features. First, it offers a rational basis for allocating health care resources for those with limited budgets. Some Canadian provinces and European countries take QALYs into account when allocating their health care dollars. Government agencies pick a threshold dollar amount and refuse to pay for any intervention whose cost per QALY exceeds it. A popular threshold is $60,000; that is, interventions that cost more than $60,000 per QALY are often deemed cost-ineffective. Interestingly, this threshold is considerably lower than the value of a year of life identified by economic studies. QALYs are slowing creeping into the U.S. health economy. The State of Oregon uses a scheme based on QALY principles for its Medicaid program, and some PBMs consider QALYs when determining whether to include certain new drugs in their formularies.

In the future, patients may be able to use QALYs to evaluate providers and health plans. It would be natural for patients to compare MCOs on the basis of QALYs gained, drawing conclusions like "Patients in HMO A gained an average of .10 QALYs last year, whereas those in HMO B gained only .07 QALYs." This would give patients a clear basis for comparing quality across plans and weighing it against cost. I imagine that some patients might be willing to pay an additional $5,000 to be in HMO A, but others might prefer to spend their money on other items. Unfortunately, such rational comparison shopping is probably a long way off. When it comes to shopping for health care, most patients remain about as well-informed as they were in the days of Marcus Welby.

ARROW REDUX

Nearly forty years after Kenneth Arrow published his seminal paper explaining why patients relied so heavily on their physicians, most patients still have a difficult time shopping for medical services. Patients may ask for drugs they see advertised on television and may question the need for surgery a bit more than they used to, but by and large they still shop the old-fashioned way. Patients ask friends and relatives for recommendations. They get referrals from their primary care physician, who rarely, if ever, looks at quality data, and they almost always follow their physician's advice. A few organizations have emerged to help patients find the "best" doctor (there are several such toll-free services in the Chicago area alone), but they usually base recommendations on admitting privileges and board certification rather than on a doctor's measured ability to effect a cure. When all is said and done, patients still do not make a serious effort to comparison shop on the basis of quality. What a risk they are taking! With mortality rates differing across providers by several percentage points, patients who do not shop for the best quality are, for all intents and purposes, playing Russian roulette.

Yet even when evidence emerges to indicate that some providers have below-average quality, most patients pretend they are in some kind of "Lake Wobegone" of medical care, where "all of the providers are above average." The *Chicago Tribune* recently published a letter to the editor concerning mortality rankings of Chicago-area hospitals that sums up how most people seem to feel about quality.[14] The letter writer, who had five children born by caesarean section, vastly preferred her hospital to higher ranked hospitals, citing the hospital's "human side." This was easy for her to say after the fact, since she and her five children beat the odds and turned out all right. If the letter writer believed the rankings, however, would she really have been willing to have her sixth child at the same hospital, knowing that this was unnecessarily dangerous? Would she have accepted even a 0.1 percent heightened mortality risk for her baby? Probably not. The "human side" is desirable, but patients deserve more than just good bedside manner. They deserve the best possible outcomes as well.

Patients will not shop around for quality unless they acknowledge that quality varies and they refuse to be treated by inferior providers. But for this to happen, patients must be able to identify the best and worst providers. This means that someone has to measure quality.

Donabedian's Trichotomy of Quality

If I could choose a single measure of outcomes quality, I would choose QALYs gained. In practice, this would mean that if I needed heart surgery, I would select the surgical team and hospital most likely to keep me alive and active for as long as possible. Taking a longer view, if I had chest pain, I would want the provider who could make the most accurate diagnosis and help me identify the best specialist if I needed one. Thinking even further ahead, if I was asymptomatic, I would want a PCP who could give me the best possible information about how to prevent heart disease. In each of these ways, I would maximize my QALYs. I think that most patients would want the same things. Right now, I have a difficult time selecting my provider because I cannot get any of this information and instead I have to rely on other measures of quality. So do most other patients.

Quality measures have been evolving for some time. Two decades ago, health services researcher Avedis Donabedian classified quality measurements in three categories: structural (or input) quality, process quality, and outcomes quality.[15] Measures of structural quality include credentialing of personnel, staffing ratios, and availability of sophisticated medical equipment. Measures of process quality include frequency of cancer screening, vaccination rates, and postoperative lengths of stay. Outcome measures include mortality, morbidity, and improvement in QALY scores. Outcome measures matter most; structure and process measures are useful largely to the extent that they are good predictors of outcomes. After all, few patients would care whether their physician went to Harvard or whether their hospital has an MRI facility unless Harvard credentials and MRIs lead to better outcomes.

Until the 1980s, quality measurement was largely restricted to structural and process measures. State licensure of hospitals depended on equipment, personnel, and safety features but not on outcomes. Similarly, the private Joint Commission on Accreditation of Hospitals, founded in 1951, based accreditation mainly on structural measures. (I recall my

Cornell professors bemoaning the emphasis placed on such "indicators of quality" as the availability of fire extinguishers.) Professional Standards Review Organizations focused almost exclusively on process. Academics have also focused on structure and process. For example, most studies comparing the quality of nonprofits and for-profits have examined staffing, technology, and lengths of stay, but not outcomes.

For all the effort made to evaluate structural and process quality, little is known about their link to outcomes. The link between structure and outcomes is likely to be tenuous. At best, licensure and accreditation protect consumers against quackery. Beyond that, consumers still have no way to distinguish the best from the worst among the overwhelming majority of providers who meet the minimum standards. There is some evidence of a link between process and outcomes. The Harvard Medical Practice Study of hospital care in New York State, for example, finds that substandard processes were responsible for more than one-fourth of all adverse inpatient events.[16] Another study of care in Veterans Administration hospitals finds that patients suffered fewer inpatient complications (the outcome) when their physicians followed protocols for diagnosis and treatment (the process).[17]

Serious efforts to rank providers on the basis of outcomes began in 1984, when HCFA published hospital mortality rates for Medicare patients. HCFA reported actual and "expected" mortality rates for every U.S. hospital. With this information, anyone with a calculator could compute the ratio of actual to expected mortality and rank hospitals from "best" to "worst." From the beginning, providers complained that the HCFA reports were unfair and inaccurate. These complaints may have sounded self-serving, but they are not without cause. Early on, HCFA failed to meaningfully measure expected mortality. As a result, many highly regarded tertiary care hospitals fared poorly in rankings. As referral hospitals for the most severely ill patients, their actual mortality rates were very high, but this was not reflected in the expected rates. Though HCFA improved its methods for predicting mortality, providers remained suspicious about the validity of the rankings. Continued resistance from providers, combined with increasing private sector reporting of mortality, led HCFA to discontinue reporting mortality rates in 1992. The HCFA mortality reports were the beginning of a quiet revolution in evaluating quality. In recent years, newspapers and magazines, health care consulting firms, and state health agencies have all released their own rankings of hospital quality, based largely on mortality data. I will describe some of these rankings, often referred to as "quality report cards," later in this chapter.

Many providers continue to protest that quality report cards are inaccurate and unfair. In one recent survey, 79 percent of physicians felt that the rankings did not adequately adjust for severity.[18] Hospitals that fare poorly in the rankings inevitably complain that they are treating the sickest patients. Joseph Berman, the former medical director at Anthem Blue Cross and Blue Shield, describes this complaint as "the Holy Writ."[19] There is no doubt that rankings are imperfect, and many good providers have been tarred with a low ranking. This not only is unfair to these providers but also might cause some of their patients to go elsewhere for care, potentially to a lower quality provider. More accurate rankings would obviously be beneficial to providers and patients. But a little economic theory and evidence suggests that as long as the current rankings bear some resemblance to the underlying truth, they can be incredibly beneficial to the health economy.

ANOTHER SPOONFUL OF THEORY

In 1992, Mark Satterthwaite and I published an article in the *RAND Journal of Economics* that describes the economics of quality in health care markets.[20] We note that provider quality varies for at least two distinct reasons.[21] First, some providers are inherently more able than others. Some are brighter, some have steadier hands, some have better training, some have better recall. Second, regardless of their inherent abilities, all providers can boost their quality by hiring more and better staff, using better equipment, and so forth. These steps are generally costly, however, and some providers may balk at the expense. For example, although safety catheters could all but assure against accidental reuse, only 15 percent of providers were willing to bear the additional expense to purchase them. (New federal rules will require all providers to use safety catheters.) These reasons for quality variation are not unique to health care. What distinguishes health care is that patients have a hard time measuring quality and, at the same time, may not care very much about price. Satterthwaite and I wanted to know what would happen if patients had better, though still imperfect, information about quality. Better information would make it easier for patients to identify the best and worst providers. Would patients change the way they shop for care? More important, how would providers respond? Would the relative absence of price shopping matter?

We were especially interested in determining how managed care fit into the equation. Given that MCOs emerged as a vehicle for cost containment, it is tempting to conclude that the focus on costs would cause providers to reduce quality. Theory offers support for this conclusion. MCOs drive down provider margins. With lower margins, providers have less incentive and ability to maintain high quality. This is analogous to the explanation for quality reductions under the Medicare PPS and Medicaid, for which there is ample empirical support.

But Satterthwaite and I develop a counterargument. MCOs have unprecedented access to data that they could use for comparison shopping, not just on the basis of cost but also on the basis of quality. MCOs could use these data to identify the best providers and steer patients to them. If they did, then high-quality providers would stand to gain managed care patients, and low-quality patients would stand to lose them. This provides an economic incentive for all providers to boost their quality that did not exist when patients and their PCPs were selecting providers. We show that with this economic incentive in place, even small improvements in measuring the quality of health care providers can lead to substantial increases in quality.

The implications of the theory for the health economy are clear. As long as quality report cards bear some resemblance to reality, they can be a boon for patients, even if they are unfair to some providers. Report cards enable patients to slowly gravitate toward better providers. More significantly, they give all providers an incentive to boost quality.

The idea that sellers will boost quality in response to consumer information about quality is hardly a revelation. To offer just one prominent example, when consumer advocates reported in the 1980s on the quality gap between American and Japanese automobiles, many Americans began buying Japanese cars. As a result, the U.S. automakers sharply improved their quality, so that even loyal U.S. car buyers benefited. Bear in mind that the U.S. automakers had no incentive to boost quality until consumers found out that they could obtain better quality elsewhere. The same lesson may well apply to health care providers. Unless and until patients discover that provider quality varies, the incentive for providers to boost quality is muted.

A Proviso (and a Rebuttal)

Providers are quick to offer a proviso. Depending on how quality is measured, providers can potentially boost their quality score by refusing to treat the most seriously ill patients. Eric Schneider and Arnold Epstein offer a good example.[22] Pennsylvania began reporting mortality scores for cardiac surgeons in 1992. The majority of cardiac surgeons responding to a survey stated that as a result of the rankings, they were less willing to operate on more severely ill patients. Once again, economic theory suggests that this is not an altogether terrible outcome. It seems likely that the providers who are most willing to take on the sickest patients are those who are best able to care for them (and therefore least likely to suffer an adverse quality score).[23] In other words, even if some providers "game" the system by refusing to treat severely ill patients, these patients themselves may be better off because they will end up under the care of more capable providers. Unfortunately, if there is enough gaming by providers, some seriously ill patients may fail to receive treatment altogether. This would be a terrible outcome, brought about by purely selfish provider behavior. As I report later in this chapter, there is some evidence that this is just what has happened in New York and Pennsylvania in the wake of these states' release of cardiac surgery report cards.

QUALITY MEASUREMENT IN PRACTICE

Outcomes-based quality measurement is deceptively simple. To compute a provider's severity-adjusted quality score, one divides the actual incidence of mortality or morbidity for that provider by the expected incidence of mortality or morbidity. The adjustment for expected incidence is critical. Without it, providers who treat the most severely ill patients will routinely appear to have the worst quality.

The Numerator

The first step in computing severity-adjusted quality is to measure the numerator, namely, mortality or morbidity. It is easy to measure mortality for Medicare patients by using Social Security Administration death records, matched to HCFA Medicare claims data. It is also possible to measure inpatient mortality rates in the twenty or so states that compile and report hospital utilization data on all patients. HCFA and several states make their data available to the public.

For most illnesses, including most that require hospitalization, mortality is extremely rare. Thus, hospital quality rankings are often limited to a few high-mortality illnesses such as heart disease. For other illnesses, there are more telling indicators of a good outcome. Depending on the illness, patients will care about whether they fully recover, whether they can resume work and other activities, whether they experience any discomfort, how long it takes to recover, and so forth. Patients undergoing prostate surgery, for example, may be very interested in comparing rates of incontinence. In the past few years, researchers have embraced a broad-based outcomes measurement tool, the SF-36 patient questionnaire. Developed by John Ware and Cathy Sherbourne, the thirty-six questions generate eight different outcomes scores, including physical functioning (such as ability to climb stairs), social functioning (such as ability to work), mental health, and bodily pain.[24] Researchers have used the SF-36 in more than 750 publications. But even though the questionnaire takes less than ten minutes to complete, providers rarely administer it (or the two-minute SF-12) to their patients. Thus, mortality remains the only broadly available outcome measure.

The Denominator

As difficult as it is to measure actual outcomes, it is even more difficult to measure expected outcomes. Perhaps this is why doing so has become a big business. Since the early 1980s, dozens of private organizations have developed proprietary prediction models with names like APACHE, MedisGroups, Body Systems Count, and Disease Staging. Most of these models use diagnostic and demographic information available from federal and state data sources to predict mortality.[25] The models combine information in different ways and report different measures. Some report probabilities of mortality for each patient; others place patients into severity categories. The organizations that have developed these various models use them for the same purpose: to rank and quantitatively score provider quality.

Patients may be familiar with some of the rankings. Every year since 1990, *U.S. News and World Report* has combined mortality data (computed last year by the Sachs Group consulting firm) with reputation scores (obtained from surveys) to identify the nation's leading hospitals. In October 1998, America's Health Network, a Florida-based cable channel and Web site, hired HCIA, another consulting firm, to rank hospitals in major metropolitan areas. In March 1999, the industry trade magazine *Modern Healthcare* reported the rankings done by the Center for Healthcare Industry Performance Studies (CHIPS), yet another consulting firm. These firms were already in the business of evaluating quality before they were tapped by these media outlets.

The Sachs Group, HCIA, and CHIPS have gone public with their rankings as a way to promote their services. Many other consulting firms, including the MEDSTAT group and MediQual Systems, produce similar rankings for anonymous clients. One set of clients is providers who might want to further probe the data to better understand their rankings and possibly retain the consulting firms to identify ways to improve quality. Another set of clients is purchasers eager to use quality (and cost) data when forming networks.

Do the Rankings Make a Difference?

Quality report cards can make a difference to the performance of a market only if consumers use them. But the evidence thus far suggests that consumers are largely ignoring report cards. A 1997 study found that hospital market shares in the early 1990s were completely unmoved by HCFA mortality rankings.[26] Indeed, market shares were much more susceptible to newspaper reports of single unexpected deaths than they were to HCFA reports of systematic mortality differences. One possible explanation is that most patients were unaware of the HCFA rankings. Many more Americans know about J. D. Powers and *Consumer Reports* rankings of automobile quality than know about HCFA or other rankings of hospital quality.

A 1998 study of how New Yorkers responded to cardiac surgery outcomes data is slightly more encouraging. The authors found that a hospital experiencing a 3 percentage point increase in reported mortality would lose roughly 5 percent of its CABG patients to other hospitals.[27] The authors suggest that this shows that report cards are effective (the study is titled "Quality of Care Information Makes a Difference"). Yet I wonder why 95 percent of the hospital's patients continue to tolerate such a nontrivial mortality risk.

The onus of learning about and responding to report cards need not rest with patients, of course. It is sufficient that their referring physicians pay attention to them. In their study of the Pennsylvania cardiac surgery mortality rankings, however, Schnieder and Epstein found that the vast majority of cardiologists ignored the rankings when making referrals.[28] This begs the question of why cardiac surgeons might refuse to treat severely ill patients. That is, why would a surgeon care about rankings if no one pays attention to them? More recent experiences in Pennsylvania reinforce the view that ignorance can render quality rankings impotent. To improve its efforts to measure and report hospital quality for heart patients, the Pennsylvania Health Care Cost Containment Council (PHC4), the state agency charged with processing and reporting hospital outcomes data, asked for help from the renowned Leonard Davis Institute (LDI) at the University of Pennsylvania. The PHC4 wanted LDI to develop state-of-the-art outcomes measures that consumers could easily interpret. LDI constructed a simple quality measure based on mortality, "major morbidities," and "complications."[29]

Although LDI used sophisticated methods and ranked every hospital in the state, PHC4 publications only identified those hospitals whose superior or inferior performances were unlikley to have been due to chance. In doing so, PHC4 put more weight on being fair to hospitals than it did on informing consumers. Objecting to the PHC4 emphasis on fairness, LDI researchers argued that this reflected an "epidemiological" model of decision making, in which medical intervention is withheld unless there is virtual statistical certainty of its need (hence the physician dictum: "do no harm").

From the perspective of trying to harness market forces, "do no harm" is the wrong prescription. In the absence of information about quality, the harm is already being done. Patients will select below-average providers roughly half the time and not even realize it. Rankings enable patients to improve their odds of finding an above-average provider and encourage all providers to boost their quality. LDI did not pretend that its rankings were perfect, but it clearly stated that "our measures indicate good bets, not sure things."

PHC4 did manage to identify several hospitals as poor performers, but there is no evidence that patients shied away from them. LDI researchers confessed that very few patients were aware of the rankings, and those who did know of them probably did not use them when selecting a hospital. LDI research team leader Mark Pauly conjectures that "patients have been so misled by decades of physician licensure and hospital accreditation, which appeared to promise that all doctors and hospitals were pretty good, that they cannot deal with information that tells them otherwise."[30] If true, the sorry result is that patients will get the quality they ask for—highly variable and rarely as good as it can be.

Other evidence suggests that Pauly is overly pessimistic. The fact that consulting firms continue to get paid a lot of money to generate rankings means that someone finds them valuable. This view is backed up by a recent Commonwealth Fund survey, in which 30 percent of employers stated that clinical outcomes were very important to them when selecting health plans.[31] Rankings are also grist for hospital marketing mills, as hospitals attempt to secure managed care contracts at favorable prices. As providers become more sophisticated in promoting their rankings, and consumers grow more accustomed to hearing about them, perhaps more employers and employees will begin to take notice.

The Good News and the Bad News

At least one 1998 study suggests that the rankings are starting to pay off for consumers. Elizabeth DeLong, Eric Peterson, and their colleagues study the impact of New York State's "cardiovascular scorecards," which rank surgeons performing coronary artery bypass surgery.[32] DeLong and Peterson find that subsequent to the introduction of the scorecards in 1990, mortality rates in New York declined by 33 percent, compared with a 19 percent decline nationwide over the same period. With this decline, New York achieved the lowest severity-adjusted mortality rate in the nation. Moreover, DeLong and Peterson find no evidence that high-risk patients were unable to obtain care, at least as evidenced by an absence of travel to out-of-state hospitals. This appears to refute the frequent claim that providers will shun high-risk patients so as to boost their quality scores.

But Dan Kessler, Mark McClellan, Mark Satterthwaite, and I offer a demoralizing rebuttal to Delong and Peterson.[33] Examining report cards in New York and Pennsylvania, we find that among patients who had acute myocardial infarction (AMI; i.e., heart attack), mortality rates slightly increased following the release of report cards. The reason? Hospitals dramatically reduced the rate of CABG surgery for the most severely ill AMI patients. Moreover, they increased the rate of surgery for relatively healthy patients. This may help explain the DeLong and Peterson finding that the mortality rate *among those receiving surgery* declined. Our findings seem to support the contention made by many providers that report cards do harm patients by making it harder for them to receive care. (Ironically, it is the providers themselves whose actions are directly responsible for the increased mortality rates.)

We offer two rays of hope for report cards. First, we note that if report cards examine mortality rates for all patients with a given disease (e.g., heart disease), rather than all patients who receive a given treatment (e.g., CABG), it would be more difficult for providers to game the system by refusing treatment. A study by Lu et al. of Maine's performance-based contracting in substance abuse treatment supports this claim.[34] Maine evaluates and rewards mental health providers based on the overall health and functioning of substance abusers, rather than outcomes for specific interventions. Lu et al. find that providers are making more appropriate referrals to treatment centers, and that compliance has increased. We also note that our AMI study examines trends only in the first few years after the release of report cards. It is possible that, over time, many hospitals will respond to report cards by making an effort to improve their quality. This is already occurring in New York, where many high-mortality hospitals revamped their cardiac surgery programs and hired new doctors in an effort to improve their scores. For example, when Erie County Medical Center had the worst mortality score in the state in the early 1990s, it replaced the director of its heart surgery program and eventually ranked among the best hospitals in the state.

Report cards are slowly finding their way into the private sector. Anthem Blue Cross and Blue Shield has been ranking hospitals based on heart surgery mortality since 1995. Anthem refuses to reimburse for heart surgery at the bottom-ranking hospitals and offers a premium payment to the top-ranking hospitals (the best of which, in a recent ranking, is across the state line in Kentucky). Since Anthem adopted this policy, the rates of mortality and other adverse outcomes from heart surgery have fallen dramatically. Perhaps this is due to provider gaming. More significantly, many of the hospitals that Anthem dropped have revamped their surgery programs in the hope of improving their rankings. The massive efforts that hospitals in New York and Ohio have undertaken to improve their rankings belie the complaint that the rankings have nothing to do with reality. These efforts also confirm the theory that even if the rankings are inaccurate, they can profoundly help consumers by giving providers incentives to boost quality. Anthem believes that its rankings will not only improve outcomes but also reduce costs, as patients endure fewer complications and readmissions.

While Anthem's efforts have been well publicized, other MCOs are also directing patients to higher quality hospitals, though with less fanfare. A research team led by Dr. José Escarce examines hospital choices of California patients requiring bypass surgery in 1994 and finds that HMO patients were more likely to be directed to high-quality hospitals (i.e., those with lower than expected mortality rates) than were non-HMO patients.[35] MCOs in other parts of the country also attempt to reward good quality. Aetna U.S. Healthcare has a plan dating back to the late 1980s that offers financial incentives to providers who fare well on chart reviews and patient satisfaction surveys. In 1996, Blue Choice HMO of St. Louis instituted a plan that rewards physicians who score highly on patient satisfaction and several objective performance measures. The link between these incentive plans and outcomes is unclear; the plans sometimes place a greater premium on good record keeping than on good patient care. Despite this concern, we can expect payers to continue to elevate the importance of quality—as they measure it—in both network design and compensation. But our findings from New York and Pennsylvania are cautionary. If payers evaluate the quality of a particular intervention rather than the treatment of a particular illness, they should expect providers to game the system. Moreover, many of the benefits of report cards may take years to materialize, as poor performers revamp the way they provide care.

Are the Rankings Any Good? Will They Get Better?

Despite fifteen years of quality report cards, there are still just a few published rankings of hospitals, and those few are based almost exclusively on mortality, with a focus on heart surgery. For the vast majority of consumers, such information is of little or no value. The lack of good data on quality is not for a want of trying. The problem is that it is remarkably difficult to do any better with the data at hand.

Mortality is a rare event for most illnesses and procedures, and many deaths are beyond the control of providers. This gives mortality lousy statistical properties when used as a benchmark for quality because the relatively large element of chance makes it difficult to develop precise rankings. Measuring quality by mortality also means that many incidents of poor outcomes go unremarked. Some of these incidents can be picked up by measures such as postoperative length of stay and surgical complication rates, and outcomes researchers are becoming increasingly sophisticated in using these alternatives. But even these measures are valuable only to the extent they are good correlates of outcomes. Unfortunately, there is no systematic measurement of nonfatal outcomes, such as the SF-36, in publicly available data. Nor have researchers developed risk adjusters to help determine if a low score on the SF-36 can be attributed to the provider or the patient. Even if such measures were available, it would be too difficult to link data across providers to identify who is responsible for poor outcomes. There are simply too many limits to what can be accomplished using available data, and it may require a coordinated effort to make substantial improvements to the data.

The Joint Commission on the Accreditation of Healthcare Organizations (JCAHO) has embarked on one such effort. As part of the accreditation process, the JCAHO requests hospitals, outpatient surgery centers, nursing homes, and other providers to identify "sentinel events," defined to be "an unexpected occurrence involving death or serious physical or psychological injury, or the risk thereof. Serious injury specifically includes loss of limb or function. The phrase, 'or the risk thereof' includes any process variation for which a recurrence would carry a significant chance of a serious adverse outcome."[36] The JCAHO has compiled a "sentinel event database" that is richer than any mortality-only database. (Note that this private sector effort predates by several years President Clinton's call for a similar database on medical mistakes.) For now, the JCAHO is mainly concerned with how organizations respond to sentinel events, and it uses information about frequency and response to sentinel events as part of its accreditation process. Consumers can search the JCAHO Web site to learn a provider's accreditation status (e.g., accredited with commendation, conditional accreditation), but the JCAHO should do more than just give accreditation status. On the theory that noisy information that is correlated with the truth is better than no information at all, the JCAHO should provide its own rankings.

The JCAHO has the clout to do this. By threatening to withhold accreditation from noncooperative hospitals (which would then face loss of payments from many payers), the JCAHO could force hospitals to provide complete data on sentinal events or other indicators of poor outcomes. It could then rank the providers or offer the data to private organizations, which would do their own rankings. The JCAHO prefers to encourage providers to respond to quality problems without pressure from the market. I suspect that market pressures, fair or unfair, will do much to hasten provider responses.

Given that so many organizations, ranging from consulting firms to the government and the JCAHO, have found it difficult to systematically measure quality, it goes without saying that it is all but impossible for individuals to do so. Few individuals can afford the data, and only a fraction of them have the statistical skills to make much sense out of them. Even the Internet is not a very helpful tool for measuring quality. No user groups or e-mail communities can provide the kind of systematic outcomes and severity data needed to construct sophisticated report cards. For now, Web surfers can find some rudimentary rankings by visiting the JCAHO, healthgrades.com, or other sites. But as these sites obtain better data and generate more accurate rankings, consumers will be able to cheaply and confidently identify the best-sellers.

RANKING MCOs

Ultimately, it may not matter whether consumers pay attention to quality rankings. If MCOs use the rankings to design networks, then market forces will work to the benefit of consumers. Most consumers do not trust their MCOs to pay attention to quality, however, and might expect MCOs to ignore quality rankings in favor of the lowest cost providers.[37] But MCOs seem to care enough about quality to include prominent teaching hospitals in their networks, despite their high cost. Maybe these hospitals lend a patina of quality to MCO networks by virtue of their brand identity in their local markets. It is one thing for MCOs to pay attention to the superficiality of brand names that appeal to patients. It is quite another for them to use actual outcomes-based quality measures, especially when consumers know so little about them.

The market does have the potential to force MCOs to provide what patients want. MCOs have expanded their networks in response to patients' concerns about access. Reports from New York, New Jersey, and other states indicate that patients almost never appeal MCO access decisions.[38] In 1997, for example, the six largest MCOs in the state averaged about 2.5 appeals per 1,000 patients, prompting observers like Alain Enthoven to wonder if MCOs are making too few denials. With patients (and legislators) expressing growing concern about access to emergency care, expect MCOs to further loosen up on access restrictions.

The facts that MCOs include teaching hospitals in their networks and pay attention to access have a common thread: patients can easily identify teaching hospitals and can easily assess access. This fits squarely with Burt Weisbrod's view that profit-making firms do not skimp on easy-to-measure attributes. But this leaves open the possibility that they will cut back on hard-to-measure attributes, which is a central concern among those who believe that profit-seeking MCOs will harm quality. Of course, one way to alleviate these concerns is to improve the measurement of MCO quality. About a decade ago, several large national employers, assisted by a few MCOs, launched an effort to do just that.

NCQA: Using Market Forces to Assure Quality

The National Committee for Quality Assurance (NCQA) was created in 1991 by several national employers, HMOs, and nonprofit foundations that wanted objective information about MCO quality. NCQA proponents believe that the best way to help patients shop for MCOs is to provide comparative data on multiple dimensions of quality. With these data, patients will not have to rely on trust to assure quality; instead, they can rely on market forces. The centerpiece of NCQA efforts is the Health Plan Employer Data and Information Set (HEDIS). Now in its fifth edition, HEDIS 2000 is completed by virtually all HMOs. To date, there is no comparable report on PPOs.

A completed HEDIS report can be over fifty pages long, with six "domains" of outcomes information, such as "effectiveness of care" (e.g., rates of immunization for children and flu shots to adults; percentage of newborns with low birth weights), use of services, (e.g., chemical dependency utilization; caesarean section rate), and member satisfaction (based on surveys). NCQA uses this information to accredit health plans and they make the full HEDIS report available to interested employers and employees. NCQA accreditation is not a rubber stamp. It is a challenge for HMOs to obtain NCQA's highest mark (full accreditation) and NCQA denies accreditation to roughly 10 percent of plans.

HEDIS seems like a managed care purchaser's dream. It is a comprehensive and hard-nosed tool for evaluating HMOs. No individual or firm could otherwise hope to obtain the wealth of information contained in HEDIS reports, and without HEDIS, individuals and firms have little hard evidence on HMO quality. Many influential employers, including Ameritech, Citibank, Digital Equipment, and IBM use HEDIS to evaluate and reward high-quality HMOs. In a recent study, Helen Schauffler, Catherine Brown, and Arnold Milstein report on the most ambitious effort to date to directly tie HMO pay to performance.[39] The Pacific Business Group on Health (PBGH) is the largest employer health care coalition in the United

States, representing nearly forty large employers (employing 3 million workers) in California. About half the members of PBGH belong to the PBGH Negotiating Alliance, which negotiates HMO premia and plan design. Beginning in 1996, the Alliance negotiated performance guarantees, whereby HMOs place 2 percent of premia at risk across a set of roughly twenty performance measures, most of which are drawn from HEDIS. Schauffler, Brown, and Milstein report that most HMOs are meeting the targets, and this has enabled the Alliance to toughen them. Due to this success, more employers have joined the Alliance. Employers elsewhere are copying the PBGH model. The U.S. Office of Personnel Management, the nation's largest employee benefits organization, is adopting a similar pay-for-performance program. General Electric, General Motors, Xerox, and the State of California (in behalf of state workers) also link HMO pay to performance. The Big Three automakers (General Motors, Ford, and Chrysler) have even combined with the United Auto Workers to develop an HMO report card based on HEDIS data.

The Trouble with HEDIS

Despite these efforts, studies show that most employers and employees have ignored HEDIS. Only 11 percent of large employers responding to a 1998 Commonwealth Fund survey stated that NCQA accreditation was "very important" in their choice of health plan.[40] Only 1 percent provided HEDIS data to their employees. And when shown HEDIS data, employees focused on member satisfaction, rather than more objective measures of quality. Such a conundrum! Most Americans do not trust their HMOs to provide quality care, yet they ignore information that might help them choose a high quality HMO.

Anyone who has looked at a full HEDIS report can readily explain why it is ignored. Once one gets beyond the final HEDIS score (accreditation), the rest of the report is difficult to read and interpret. NCQA intends HEDIS to be a scorecard for MCOs. Most scorecards keep a single score for each "team." But a typical HEDIS report contains hundreds of "scores," with dozens of statistics within each measurement domain. Someone reading a HEDIS report on their own managed care plan may discover that providers in the plan advised 61 percent of its smoking members to quit, that the average length of stay for newborns is 1.59 days, and that the plan had a ratio of cash to claims payable of 3.1. They would find statistics on dozens of other dimensions. But so what? This is information without content. No wonder that employees skip all these details and just focus on member satisfaction. At least this is a single score that is easy to interpret.

In the past year, the NCQA has taken dramatic steps to make HEDIS more user friendly. The NCQA takes HEDIS responses and constructs

Health Plan Report Cards. These report cards give plans one to four stars on five dimensions of performance:

1. Access and service (e.g., number of contracting providers; ease of scheduling appointments)

2. Provider quality (based on credentials and consumer surveys)

3. Health maintenance (e.g., do patients receive appropriate diagnostic tests)

4. Getting better (e.g.,availability of up-to-date treatment technologies)

5. Living with illness (e.g., does the HMO have plans to assist patients with chronic illnesses?)

Patients can easily obtain these rankings from the NCQA Web site.

It remains to be seen whether employers and employees will embrace this new ranking system. It is not without some serious flaws. One major problem is that most plans within a given metropolitan area receive very similar rankings. This is no surprise, as many HEDIS scores depend on provider performance, and most plans in a given market have similar provider networks. Another problem is that some rankings, such as those based on utilization and patient compliance, depend as much on the performance of patients as on the performance of the HMOs.

Perhaps the biggest problem with HEDIS is that it does not directly measure outcomes quality. Certainly some of the process indicators are correlated with outcomes, but these represent the tip of the quality iceberg. Consider that Anthem gets no credit in the HEDIS scorecard for its efforts to steer patients to the best cardiac surgery providers, and could lose marks if broader steering causes patients to have to wait for certain services. For all of its domains of measurement, HEDIS measures seem to ignore the most important questions about the quality of MCOs. Does plan X's utilization review program cost lives? What about plan Y's restriction on access to specialists, or plan Z's stingy capitation rates? Do they remove the fat from the health care system, or do they cut into the lean? HEDIS provides no answers.

Patients will not fully hold MCOs accountable for quality until they have answers to these questions. But this will require better data, and a willingness of both providers and consumers to change the way they think about quality. In the final chapter, I identify some of the steps that must be taken to make this happen.

CHAPTER 8

Fulfilling the Promise of Managed Care

THROUGHOUT the evolution of the health economy, it has remained difficult for patients to efficiently and effectively shop for health care goods and services. The defining features of the health economy—from trust, physician autonomy, and nonprofit hospitals to selective contracting, capitation, and utilization review—are all efforts to solve the shopping problem. It is widely perceived that the managed care solution to the shopping problem emphasizes cost containment at the expense of quality. But with MCO premiums increasing by 6 to 8 percent in each of the last two years, there is growing concern that MCOs may no longer be able to contain costs.

MCOs face mounting cost pressures from several directions. Employers and employees demand ever greater access, which necessarily forces MCOs to pay more to providers. Provider and purchaser consolidation has further reduced MCO purchasing power. Perhaps most significantly, the pace of technological innovation has increased. There are new and costly treatments for seemingly every disease. Many MCOs are experiencing 15 to 20 percent annual increases in the cost of drugs alone and are passing these cost increases on to consumers.

If no one likes MCOs, and they appear to be losing their ability to control costs, why tolerate them? The answer is that MCOs should not be judged on how well they contain costs but on how well they solve the shopping problem. If MCOs do little more than use selective contracting to secure provider discounts, the MCO "solution" reduces to an administratively costly version of regulatory solutions such as the Medicare PPS. But if MCOs can use innovative incentives and new health information technologies to eliminate inefficient purchases, force providers to rationalize the adoption of new technologies, steer patients to the best and most cost-effective providers, and develop the wisest treatment plans, they are serving consumers well, regardless of the cost. What matters is not how much we spend on health care but whether we spend it wisely.

MCOs have demonstrated that competition can be a force for positive change in the health economy. But much remains to be done to assure that we achieve the goal of getting the greatest value for our health care dollars. The burden falls in various ways on all participants in the health economy—MCOs, providers, employers, the government, and patients.

IT SEEMS OBVIOUS, BUT . . .

Competitive solutions require competition. Competitive markets work when shoppers play one seller off against another and reward those who offer the best value. Shoppers not only get good quality at a reasonable price but also force sellers to be efficient and innovative. Health care is not exempt from these dynamics, and managed care enables patients to be effective shoppers. But many providers are trying to eliminate competition. If they succeed, they may well kill off managed care.

The consolidation wave in health care is a direct response to the growth of managed care.[1] Providers claim that they need to merge to become more efficient, but systematic research shows that most mergers do not generate substantial efficiencies. On the other hand, many mergers appear to reduce competition and seriously hamper MCO efforts to shop for the best value. Research that is sure to emerge in the next few years will determine whether these mergers led to higher costs.

Hospitals at least put up the pretense of efficiencies to justify their mergers (and some mergers have yielded significant savings). Physicians, on the other hand, do not hide their desire to counter MCO purchasing power. Physicians in several markets have formed organizations to facilitate colluding on price. Blocked by antitrust enforcers, they have sought to find legal ways to raise prices. They have merged into large groups that are immune to antitrust. More significantly, they are on the verge of forming unions that may also be exempt from antitrust statutes.

Under U.S. labor laws, only employees may unionize. Most physicians own their own practices and so are prohibited from unionization. Congress has considered legislation that would relax this prohibition. Through a union, physicians could collectively bargain with MCOs, which would help them to coordinate the development of guidelines and resolve disputes regarding utilization review. But paramount in the eyes of many who advocate physician unions would be their ability to command higher fees from MCOs. Physicians who defend the union movement point out that other highly trained workers are unionized. But physicians are different. Some highly trained unionized workers, such as air traffic controllers, do not work directly as agents for consumers. Those who do, such as plumbers and electricians, do not command the same trust as do physicians. Physicians also claim that their unions will not go on strike, but without the threat of a job action like a strike or a serious work slowdown, it seems unlikely that unions will be able to extract major concessions from MCOs. By taking a job action for higher fees, physicians would eliminate any pretense of being perfect agents for their patients.

Led mainly by physicians, providers are seeking other forms of legislative relief from the burdens of competition. State "any willing provider" statutes blunt competitive pressures on providers to lower their prices. These statutes enable providers to enter into MCO networks by matching the prices set by their competitors. As a result, providers have no incentive to reduce their prices. State "patient bill of rights" laws also stifle competition by preventing MCOs from excluding providers from networks. For the past five years, physicians have lobbied Congress for blanket antitrust immunity, currently through H.R. 1304, the Quality Health-Care Coalition Act of 1999. This curiously titled bill would permit physicians to fix prices by engaging in what would otherwise be blatantly criminal acts. Representative Thomas Campbell of California introduced the bill into several sessions of Congress. The U.S. House of Representatives passed the bill in June 2000, perhaps to cash in on the public's dissatisfaction with managed care. But the bill lacks a champion in the Senate, federal antitrust agencies oppose it, and President Clinton has not endorsed it, so it seems unlikely to gain passage anytime soon. However, Texas has enacted similar legislation and other states may soon follow suit.

Physicians claim that they need antitrust relief to form large, quasi-independent networks that can boost quality. This is a red herring. Physicians did not attempt to form such quality-enhancing networks prior to the growth of managed care. Besides, current antitrust rules permit physicians to create networks if they implement the kind of clinical integration needed to improve quality. The government has approved roughly 90 percent of applications to form such networks and has even approved a few networks that would allow physicians to monopolize a particular specialty in their community. Even so, few physicians have participated in those efforts to enhance quality. The inescapable truth is that physicians want Congress to enact H.R. 1304 so that they can avoid competition.

Should We Turn Back the Clock?

Patients have already witnessed a time when providers were immune to normal competitive pressures. It was not a pretty sight. Competition, to the extent it existed, involved a costly medical arms race. Inefficiency was rampant, and providers routinely offered services on the flat of the curve. Efforts to measure and reward quality were virtually nonexistent. To rein in runaway inflation, the government launched an ineffective planning effort, which gave way to managed care. Providers may claim that they will strive for efficiency and innovation, even if there is no managed care. But in the absence of aggressive shopping by MCOs, why would they? If the past is prologue, only one conclusion is possible. If providers are permitted the luxury of avoiding competition, patients should expect a return to the profligate spending of the 1960s and 1970s.

I wonder if patients have thought about what it would cost if managed care were to disappear. The odds are that the cost would be far greater than most patients have reckoned. At the start of the 1990s, before MCOs took over, private sector health care spending was rising by more than 10 percent annually, and many experts predicted health care would account for 20 percent of the GDP by the year 2000. As recently as 1993, a Congressional Budget Office report pegged that figure at 18.9 percent. Thanks to MCOs, private sector health care spending rose at 5 percent annually during the 1990s, and total spending on health care remains below 14 percent of GDP. Because of managed care, the 1993 Congressional Budget Office report overstated year 2000 spending by $300 billion. It is safe to conclude that were it not for the growth of managed care, projections that health care would represent 20 percent of GDP would not be too far off the mark.

What makes the cost savings even more noteworthy is that they have been confined almost entirely to the private sector. Medicare spending grew at twice the rate of private sector spending during the 1990s. Although a growing number of Medicare enrollees have joined HMOs, Medicare remains largely an indemnity program because HCFA still does not provide substantial incentives for MCOs to sign up Medicare enrollees or for Medicare recipients to join MCOs. If HCFA were to fully embrace managed care, total annual health care savings might exceed $500 billion.

It is remarkable to think that MCOs have reduced health care's share of GDP by nearly $300 billion annually—or close to $2,000 per privately insured patient—without any apparent systematic reduction in quality. Are patients really willing to sacrifice $2,000 annually just to restore complete decision-making power to medical providers, especially knowing that the quality of care would be largely unaffected? The market test suggests that very few would be willing to do so; indemnity insurance is still available, but no one wants to buy it. The reality is that patients want unfettered decision making for themselves and their providers, and lower medical costs for everyone. In other words, they want the proverbial free lunch.

There Is an Old Saying

Be careful what you wish for, because you might get it. The saying applies especially well to medical providers. If providers do regain power, it seems likely that MCOs, as we know them, will gradually disappear. Consider that MCOs grew in popularity by offering employers substantial savings over traditional indemnity plans. This explains why MCO penetration is largest in those markets where there is extensive provider competition—it is in these markets that MCOs drive the hardest bargains with providers and offer employers the largest savings.[2] Take away provider competition, and you take away MCOs. But that would not be the end of the story. Take away MCOs, and health care spending will start to rise once gain. Facing rising health care costs, the nation will look for solutions. With no market-based solution to turn to, the federal government would have to step in.

Many policy makers are eager to enact some form of national health insurance. If health care inflation heats up, this topic will once again take center stage in the political arena. Legislators who support national health insurance undoubtedly realize that managed care is all that stands in the way of "success"; any legislation that thwarts managed care moves them one step closer to enacting a national insurance plan. But providers who are so scornful of managed care should not rejoice at this prospect. Given the federal government's track record of ever-declining reimbursements for Medicare and Medicaid, even monopoly providers would feel the tightening of the financial screws if national health insurance should come to pass.

The logic is inescapable. Providers seek to thwart managed care through mergers, unions, and legislative relief. This will enable them to avoid competition, with the inevitable result that rapid cost increases will return to the health economy. This would surely be followed by the heavy hand of regulation. Patients and providers would all be worse off. And everyone would know where to point the finger—at the providers who demanded complete control over the system and drove it to bankruptcy.

THE NEED FOR BETTER DATA AND BETTER DATA USERS

It hardly breaks new ground to call for better health care data. For decades, various government programs have tried to unify the way that providers report cost and utilization data. The Health Systems Agencies created by the 1974 National Health Planning and Resources Development Act generated data on physician practice patterns to facilitate quality evaluation. One of the goals of the Clinton health care reform plan of 1993 was to require regional health plans to prepare "annual performance reports" to "measure how their health plans, doctors, and hospitals perform on a set of four critical indicators: Access; Appropriateness; Outcome; and Consumer Satisfaction."[3] Today, NCQA, JCAHO, consulting firms, accounting firms, and countless other health care and affiliated organizations are banking on the value of better data.

Good data have many virtues. They enable payers and providers to assess, develop, and implement innovative payment schemes. They enable capitated PCPs to do a better job of identifying efficient specialists and hospitals for referrals. Good data permit the development of norms of care that can be finely tailored to meet patients' idiosyncratic needs. Good data enable payers and providers to develop and evaluate disease management programs, and they enable patients to do a better job of identifying high-quality providers and MCOs. Ongoing efforts to generate useful data have been spotty, however, and much more needs to be done. Nearly a decade has passed since HCFA last published its hospital mortality reports, and only a few states have filled the void. In the meantime, a few private organizations have published their own lists of the best and worst providers. NCQA and healthgrades.com even post their ratings on the Internet. But the evidence suggests that patients generally ignore such objective data. This might be all right if their MCOs paid attention to provider quality when assembling networks. But MCOs are under no market pressure to do so. After all, patients almost completely ignore objective data about MCOs, including HEDIS data. It is highly implausible that patients will pay attention to whether their MCOs use report card data. If patients do not force their MCOs to look at report cards, it is the responsibility of patients to evaluate provider quality themselves. If they do not, the possibility of harnessing market forces to improve quality is lost.

Are the Data Useful?

Systematic quality measurement requires a lot of data, uniformly collected from all providers. Most states collect hospital administrative claims data (i.e., the type of data in a medical bill, such as the hospital's identity, procedures performed, diagnoses, limited demographic information, and whether the patient survived the hospital stay). Medicare also collects administrative claims data for all inpatient and outpatient services. Medicare data can be tied to national death data to measure posthospitalization mortality. Such data form the foundation for most report cards. Claims data are not ideal for quality measurement, largely because there is scant clinical information. New York and Pennsylvania supplemented claims data with some basic clinical data obtained from chart review. All states should generate similar rankings and publicize them or should follow Medicare's lead and permit private sector organizations to purchase the data and construct independent rankings.

Such rankings would be very helpful for patients who need services such as cardiac surgery, for which the mortality rate can be nontrivial. But patients with AIDS, diabetes, asthma, depression, and countless other conditions will get little use out of data on hospital utilization and posthospitalization mortality. To evaluate the quality of care for these patients, it is essential to collect more detailed outcomes data from hospitals and other providers. NCQA has started in this direction by requiring HMOs serving Medicare enrollees to provide SF-36 survey data.[4] Better still, physicians or health plans could administer the SF-36 to all their patients, perhaps during annual checkups. Patients undergoing treatment for specific conditions could also receive shorter, targeted instruments. Consumers are willing to spend considerable time completing quality surveys, as evidenced by the thousands of new-car buyers who fill out the J. D. Powers survey (which takes thirty minutes or more to complete). So it is conceivable that patients would be willing to complete an annual ten-minute outcomes survey.

These survey instruments will be of limited usefulness until researchers can get better risk adjusters. The clinical and demographic information in administrative claims data does not enable researchers to confidently attribute poor outcomes to low provider quality, and it may encourage providers to avoid treating the most severely ill patients. Better risk adjustment requires clinical data contained in medical records. More and more providers are using electronic medical records, so the technology for linking medical records to outcomes should not be an obstacle to performing meaningful outcomes research. Confidentiality would.

The Confidentiality Problem

Good outcomes research requires an electronic medical record reporting each patient's clinical condition and health status throughout the course of treatment. Creating electronic records will require two steps. First, providers must report clinical and outcomes data on electronic documents. This can be time-consuming, so someone will have to bear the expense. But good outcomes data can be enormously valuable. Payers, providers, and patients should all be willing to bear the additional expense of data generation to reap the rewards of more cost-effective medical care (though it may require some kind of private agreement or government regulation to prevent those payers or providers who do not want to bear the cost from free riding on those who do).

Second, these data must be linked across providers. To facilitate linkage, providers will have to report data in a consistent format. More important, linking data requires some way to determine whose information is being linked. In other words, linkage will require a unique patient identifier or "health care ID," akin to a Social Security number. This raises obvious concerns about confidentiality. Insurers and employers who access this ID could use it to create a comprehensive patient medical record. Most Americans oppose granting widespread access to their medical records; in fact, in one recent survey, 85 percent of respondents favored federal laws to protect the privacy of such records.[5]

Patients have some reason to seek such protection. Insurers might use the information contained in medical records for medical underwriting, while employers might use it to make decisions about hiring, promotions, and layoffs. Fearful of how the information will be used, physicians might not truthfully report diagnoses, and patients might not truthfully report their health status, compromising the validity of the data and possibly endangering patients. But patients seem unwilling to give up privacy even to groups that might use the information to advance the public health. For example, 60 percent of the respondents to the aforementioned survey would not grant access to their medical records to hospitals offering preventive care programs.

I believe that there is less to fear than meets the eye. Existing administrative claims data already contain enough clinical information to enable employers and insurers to identify patients with specific "undesirable" diseases. Yet there have been no obvious abuses of these data when they are used to measure outcomes, generate report cards, and construct disease management programs. The reason is simple: researchers engaged in these activities do not need to know the identities of patients; they are content to work with anonymous numerical identifiers. Even so, most patients want as near as possible to a guarantee that their records will remain confidential. Public and private sector efforts are under way to facilitate data linkage without divulging patient identities. Just as the AHRQ is coordinating the development of data-driven disease management programs, there is a role for the government in coordinating the development of these massive databases. There will always be doubters who fear that any form of a patient ID would lead to abuse, and there is probably no way to be absolutely certain that such abuses will not occur. But the stakes are high, and the doubters must not win out without a trial run. If there is no patient identifier, data cannot be linked. If the data are not linked, outcomes research will be stymied. And if outcomes research is stymied, efforts to promote competition among providers and MCOs on the basis of quality, and not just cost, will also be stymied.

The Law of Large Numbers

From a statistical standpoint, it is relatively easy to measure outcomes of hospital treatment because hospitals treat many patients, and therefore generate lots of data. According to the law of large numbers, the reliability of outcomes measures like mortality increases with the size of the sample used to generate them. For example, a research team led by Timothy

Hofer concludes that a physician would need to treat at least one hundred patients with diabetes for researchers to obtain reliable outcomes measures.[6] But few PCPs have more than sixty diabetes patients under their care. If the market demands that physicians generate usable outcomes data, then physicians will find it valuable to merge into larger, single-specialty groups. If the group members have similar abilities, the group can report a single, reliable measure of its quality. Of course, many physicians will want to join groups in which they are the worst member, thereby gaining from the overall strong reputation of the group; the best physicians would presumably guard against this. What we already observe to some extent among academic medical centers—where the best researchers are clustered in the top schools—would become common among groups of practitioners.

Cost Measurement

Promoting cost-effective health care requires accurate cost measurement. Payers, PHOs, and physician groups need better cost data to design and evaluate compensation systems, and individual hospitals and doctors need better cost data to determine how best to respond. Payers and providers need better cost data to develop treatment guidelines and disease management programs. Hospitals are slowly adopting activity-based cost accounting, and as more catch on, accounting firms will move down the learning curve, refine their techniques, and offer more attractive ABC products to all hospitals.

Improving cost measurement at physician offices and elsewhere in the health economy is another story. Developing and implementing cost accounting systems is expensive. Hospitals can afford the six-figure price tag, but physicians and other providers lack the financial wherewithal and have many fewer patients over whom to spread the cost. Perhaps there is a role for the federal government to subsidize the substantial up-front investment in developing cost-accounting systems. Once these systems are standardized, the cost to individual providers should come down. Providers will then be able to accurately measure their own costs. Perhaps more important, independent researchers will be able to perform accurate cost-effectiveness studies.

The Need for Better Data Users

No matter how accurately researchers measure outcomes and costs, the value of these data is greatly reduced if patients ignore them. Yet when it comes to outcomes-based report cards, that is exactly what patients are doing. Presented with data suggesting that their provider is actually second-rate, most patients respond like the letter writer to the *Chicago Tribune* mentioned in Chapter 7—they dismiss the data out of hand. This creates two problems. First, it makes it difficult for better providers and MCOs to attract more patients, while allowing poor providers and MCOs to continue to thrive. Second, it blunts the financial incentives of providers and MCOs to boost quality. How frustrating it must be for organizations that demonstrably improve quality, only to have the market fail to take notice! This is especially challenging to low-cost organizations, such as the Kaiser Foundation Health Plans, that tend to score well on objective outcomes measures yet are still considered by many to have subpar quality.

It may seem difficult to comprehend such willful indifference to objective information, especially given the often substantial variation in provider quality. But I believe that this indifference makes sense when considered in the context of *Bayesian statistics*. Most people are "Bayesian" decision makers; that is, they evaluate options by combining their priors (beliefs based on past experience) with new information. They do not necessarily give equal weight to the priors and the new information, and instead will give more credence to the one they believe is more accurate. For example, a maternity patient who has had good personal experiences with a hospital may have strong priors about that hospital's quality. Unless published rankings of hospital quality are extremely persuasive, she is unlikely to substantially update her prior beliefs about her favorite hospital. For now, most patients are not persuaded by current rankings: a few may understand their statistical limitations; others have heard providers complain about the rankings; still others are probably clueless about what the rankings mean. As long as they have reason to doubt the rankings, patients will stick to their priors.

As a prerequisite for patients to accept the rankings, providers should acknowledge that quality really does vary and that it is possible to rank quality, albeit with some error. Flawed rankings may be unfair to some providers and may encourage providers to ignore seriously ill patients. But in all other respects, even flawed rankings make for a vastly superior market. More often than not, rankings help patients find the best providers. In the long run, providers respond to rankings by boosting their quality. This raises the quality of care for all patients. Unfortunately, providers continue to view those who would evaluate quality as the enemy. For example, when the Cleveland Clinic failed to dominate the rankings of Cleveland Health Quality Choice program (CHQC), an employer-sponsored quality ranking in its local market, it criticized the methods. When CHQC recomputed the rankings to better conform with the Cleveland Clinic's wishes, they did not substantially change. The Cleveland Clinic's response was to withhold data necessary to perform the rankings. The quality-ranking project died shortly thereafter.

Once providers acknowledge that quality varies, patients will be more likely to accept the possibility that their preferred providers are below average. The increased use of the Internet is likely to speed this process along. A growing number of patients spend considerable time researching their illnesses on the Internet, often discovering a range of treatment options that do not always coincide with their own physicians' recommendations. Patients are challenging their physicians' decisions and in the process are stripping away the myth that their physicians can do no wrong. At the same time, patients are learning that medicine is not a settled science. Once they have opened their eyes to the possibility that some providers may have better answers than others, they will be more willing to seek out the best providers.

Good Shopping and Equity

In almost every product and service market, such as automobiles and law, consumers are willing to pay more to get better quality. Once patients learn to identify the best providers, the same is likely to be true in health care markets. The best providers might respond by raising their prices; those that do not will have to find some other way to ration the expected increase in demand. At the same time, lower quality providers will experience a decrease in demand, which might force them to lower their prices or specialize in easier cases. This raises the possibility that wealthier patients will have greater access to the best providers. Of course, some physicians have always charged higher prices and catered to a wealthier clientele. Physicians on Madison Avenue usually charge much more than physicians in Harlem. Few people complain that this is unfair, because while the "tonier" physicians may offer plusher waiting rooms and shorter waiting times, it is not obvious that they offer better medical care. But issues of fairness are bound to emerge as it becomes reasonably clear that wealth buys a better chance of survival, and not just leather sofas and newer magazines in the waiting room.

THE ROLE OF THE EMPLOYER

Before employees can select their managed care plan, their employer must whittle down the dozens of offerings to a handful, or maybe even just one. Employees cannot select a high-quality MCO unless their employer offers it. While many larger employers say that they consider HEDIS when selecting a plan, many others do not. Smaller employers rarely examine HEDIS. For all of HEDIS's shortcomings, it is still the best available measure of MCO quality. It is safe to conclude that many employers do not make a serious effort to evaluate plan quality. This is unfortunate, because employers are perfectly positioned to shop for MCOs. As NCQA, the various regional Business Groups on Health, the U.S. Office of Personnel Management, and Twin Cities companies have shown, employers have the purchasing clout to catch the attention of insurers, especially when they act collectively. At a minimum, they can command deep discounts. But they can also force MCOs to report a variety of quality measures and reward those MCOs that create the most value for their employees. The PBGH has even instituted a program whereby MCOs provide data on the treatment of several diseases, including breast cancer and diabetes, with the goal of establishing comprehensive databases that can be used to establish state-of-the-art disease management programs.

Employers have the wherewithal and market clout to serve as perfect agents for their employees, selecting the plans that best balance quality and cost. But the same factors that make it difficult for employees to select a health plan on their own—the lack of data and analytical expertise— make it difficult for employees to determine if their employer has done a good job in their behalf. Some employers, such as the members of NCQA, believe that it is good business practice to reward high quality MCOs, both to maintain employee health and to build employee satisfaction. These employers do not need prodding from their employees to care about MCO quality. Not all employers are so "enlightened," however. Some may seek out the lowest cost plan regardless of quality, and hope that their employees do not know it.

It is imperative that employees spend more time evaluating their MCO options. This is starting to happen, as employers introduce *defined contribution* health benefits. In a defined contribution plan, employers cover the costs of inexpensive plans, and require employees to pay the premium differential for more generous plans. Defined contribution plans make economic sense to the extent that they simultaneously give employees a choice of plans and force them to bear the full cost (actually, the after-tax cost) of generous health plans. But they run the risk of promoting adverse selection, whereby healthier patients cluster into inexpensive plans, driving up the costs for sicker patients who prefer more generous coverage. Moreover, defined contribution plans do nothing to assure that patients will pay attention to quality. Given current concerns about MCO quality, one would think that it would take very little to arouse such interest. Consider that the cost of a typical sports utility vehicle expected to last five years is about the same as the cost of five years of family health insurance coverage. Yet few employees spend as much time comparing MCO quality as they do comparing automobile and SUV quality. Perhaps HEDIS reports are indecipherable. But NCQA ratings have become more user friendly, and employees can also turn to ratings in *Consumer Reports* and other outlets. I suspect that if employees use these ratings, more and better ratings will emerge. Employees owe it to themselves to make at least a small effort to validate their employer's choice of MCO.

WHAT DOES MCO REALLY STAND FOR?

It is not outlandish to claim that if all the aforementioned objectives are met (better data, provider buy-in to report cards, informed patients), then MCOs need only be good competitors to best serve the interests of enrollees. Those that fail to deliver value to their enrollees will lose out in the competitive market. Or will they? One need only look at the MCO track record to date to be skeptical. Most MCOs seem to have succeeded by following a few simple strategies, mainly selective contracting and UR. Selective contracting is the low-hanging fruit of managed care. It has been relatively easy for MCOs to dangle "covered lives" in front of providers, secure discounts, and use those discounts to obtain a few employer contracts. But selective contracting solely for the sake of obtaining discounts is a way to "manage prices," not manage care, and some critics claim derisively that MCO stands for "managed *cost* organization."

MCOs that survive solely by negotiating price discounts preserve the same inefficiencies associated with flat-of-the-curve medicine, practice variations, and so forth. They do not direct patients to the best providers or encourage providers to find better ways to deliver care. For all the savings that selective contracting generates, when MCOs rely solely on obtaining discounted prices, most of the potential of managed care to improve the delivery of health care remains untapped. If MCOs do not evolve beyond discounting, perhaps patients might be better off under a single-payer system in which the government achieves lower costs by dictating price reductions. At least in such a system there would be no marketing expenses, no medical underwriting, and full, portable insurance.

The focus on obtaining discounts has motivated the current MCO merger wave and resurrected the fear that the health economy will one day be dominated by a handful of investor-owned firms. This time, there is a sound economic logic underlying the fear. While MCO mergers do not create substantial operating efficiencies, they do permit MCOs to realize even deeper discounts. The most recent spate of MCO mergers has motivated physicians and hospitals to seek countervailing market power, creating the troubling prospect of a monopoly MCO dealing with a cartel of physicians and a monopoly hospital system. If the health economy ever gets to that point, then innovation and efficiency would surely be replaced by negotiation, power plays, and lobbying for legislation. Antitrust agencies should block MCO mergers not because they threaten the livelihoods of physicians but because they threaten the future of managed care.

Can MCOs Survive?

MCOs complain that if they do not consolidate, market forces will drive them out of business. Some consolidation does seem inevitable. As long as MCOs pursue the same strategies, they will be unable to build consumer loyalty, and price competition will remain fierce. Once a few MCOs exit (and, equally important, fewer MCOs enter), competition should ease, allowing the remaining MCOs to raise premiums by enough to remain viable.

Most MCOs are unwilling to wait for the shakeout, perhaps fearful that they will be the next to exit. MCOs can avoid competition through merger, but this solution is unlikely to serve enrollees very well. Instead, MCOs will need to differentiate themselves to survive. Oxford Health appeared on the verge of creating a "top-quality" HMO when poor accounting sent it into bankruptcy. But as more patients use better data, such opportunities for differentiation will increase. High-quality MCOs will be able to attract more patients and command higher premiums. MCOs can help make this happen by facilitating quality evaluation. They can require their physicians to administer the SF-36, or review medical records to construct enrollee QALY scores. They can then permit independent organizations to use this information to rank the MCOs.

MCOs can also serve the public interest by permitting independent organizations to use claims data in cost-effectiveness research. Better still, they can permit researchers to merge data across MCOs to create longitudinal databases on patient care rather than rely on mergers to create large databases. This will allow MCOs and providers to obtain the kind of detailed data necessary to advance the development and evaluation of disease management programs without unnecessarily increasing MCO market power.

MARCUS WELBY AND ASSOCIATES

Through all the changes that have taken place in the health economy, the primary care physician remains firmly at the center. HMOs still require enrollees to select a PCP, require the PCPs to make referrals to specialists, and rely on capitated payments to PCPs to limit unnecessary utilization.

If anything, the growth of managed care has increased the demand for PCPs and has given them control over both medical decision making and financing. PCPs have unprecedented opportunities to help solve their patients' shopping problems. This will not be easy. PCPs must keep abreast of technological change while also mastering the new information technologies. They must be able to evaluate and advise their patients on drug therapies, treatment protocols, and disease management programs. They must be able to evaluate and recommend MCOs and pass judgment on report cards.

If PCPs do not provide the information, others will do so. Witness the many advertisements for new drugs, hospital centers of excellence, and MCOs. These ads enable organizations that have no agency relationship with patients to attempt to influence medical decision making. The ads are effective, in part, because they fill an information vacuum; without them, patients would get no information at all about many of these drugs, providers, and MCOs. It remains to be seen whether well-informed input from PCPs will hold more sway than information offered up by Madison Avenue. Moving beyond the battle with advertisers, there are many other medical goods and services that are rarely, if ever, advertised to patients. PCPs must be aware of these as well so that they can recommend those that best meet their patients' needs.

Experts at Finding Experts

When their patients require hospitalization or the attention of specialists, PCPs must become experts at finding experts. Rather than bemoan the possibility of developing perfect provider report cards, PCPs should welcome the emphasis on quality that accompanies the publication of even imperfect rankings. A good start would be for PCPs to make sense of available report cards. Few patients will have the statistical expertise to fully appreciate the strengths and weaknesses of various report cards, but there is no reason for providers to be ignorant. As rankings become more commonplace, patients are sure to ask their PCPs why their favorite hospital or doctor is not at the top of the list. PCPs owes their patients a better response than "the rankings do not mean anything."

To prepare PCPs for the task, medical schools and residency training programs should beef up preparation in statistics and data analysis. This would also enable PCPs to do a better job of keeping up with the medical literature, evaluating claims by drug makers, and comparing treatment guidelines. By carefully evaluating HEDIS reports and other MCO quality rankings, PCPs should even be able to help patients select their MCO. The challenge of developing both clinical and statistical expertise about illnesses, providers, and MCOs will overwhelm any one PCP. We can expect PCPs to form groups, divide up research responsibilities, and share their knowledge among all group members. In this way, Marcus Welby, solo practitioner, will be replaced by Marcus Welby and Associates. The group will collectively take on the responsibility of helping patients solve the shopping problem. How will patients identify the best "shoppers?" To some extent, they will have to rely on trust, just as they always have when selecting a PCP. Larger groups may be able to present evidence about their performance, but this will require the kinds of advances in data collection outlined earlier.

Getting Paid to Shop

The most important task of the PCP is, as ever, to solve the shopping problem. Yet PCPs do not normally charge for performing this service. In most cases, PCPs and other physicians bill insurers for procedures, as spelled out by the current procedural terminology (CPT) code. The CPT codes whose descriptions come closest to "helping patients shop for medical services" are the ones for routine office visits and case management. Though enormously valuable to patients, these are among the least remunerative of all "procedures." Physicians who are capitated receive nothing for solving the shopping problem and can even lose money by making referrals. Facing low CPT-based and capitation payments, physicians have a strong economic incentive to churn their patients, seeing as many patients as possible in a given amount of time. This necessarily means less time to shop and, more critically, less time to do the research and analysis necessary to be a good shopper. This was not so important thirty years ago, when there was not much information available for PCPs to research and analyze. It is of vital importance today.

In the current economic environment, if patients want their physicians to be expert shoppers, they will have to demand it and pay for it. I can imagine two payment models. A "fee-per-advice" model would resemble existing fee-for-service payments. A "retainer" model would resemble capitation. To promote shopping under the retainer model, patients would explicitly reward physicians who provide good advice with continued business and higher retainer fees. If insurers will not boost fees, then either patients or their employers must do so. It remains to be seen whether patients will be willing to pay the price necessary to obtain expert shopping. But with MCO premiums running at around $5,000 or more for family plans, many employees might be willing to pay a few hundred dollars to obtain expert help in making sure they are getting their money's worth.

SOLVING THE SHOPPING PROBLEM

The evolution from Marcus Welby to managed care, interrupted by a brief experiment with planning, did not happen by accident. Instead, it occurred because patients had grown frustrated with rising health care costs and perceived that they were not getting good value for their health care dollars. As the health economy has expanded and grown more complex, the level of frustration has increased. As a result, most patients seem to yearn for the traditional solution to the shopping problem, in which physicians once again take total control of the health economy. Patients may remember how reassuring it was to have their trusted physicians in charge of the system, but thus apparently have forgotten (or never acknowledged in the first place) that Marcus Welby medicine was fraught with inefficiency and failed to assure quality.

At least during the heyday of Marcus Welby medicine, patients had an excuse to delegate all decision-making authority to their physicians. At that time, patients had little reason to believe that there was "immense" variation in the quality of providers. Even if they held this belief, they had little information to help them locate the best providers. Nor was there any reason for patients to shop around to find the best health plans—aside from copayment and premiums, insurance plans were all pretty much the same.

There is no longer any reason to return to Marcus Welby medicine. Sure, it is possible to improve the old system around the margins, perhaps by imposing larger copayments and deductibles. Such changes might eliminate some moral hazard utilization, but they would do little to reduce inducement and practice variations, promote price competition, facilitate quality shopping, or motivate providers to stay innovative and efficient. But the rise of managed care, combined with the ongoing revolution in health information technologies, offers patients an unprecedented opportunity to solve these problems. Selective contracting enables MCOs to get better prices from providers. Outcomes research enables MCOs and providers to identify the most cost-effective ways to treat and manage disease. Report cards help patients identify some of the best and worst MCOs and providers. These new solutions to the shopping problem are moving the health economy toward an ideal combination of low prices, efficient production, and high quality—in other words, value maximization.

I am optimistic that the health economy will reach this goal of value maximization and that MCOs will continue to play an important part. American consumers are very good about demanding value. If markets remain competitive, and purchasers—MCOs and patients alike—have the information they need to make informed choices, those organizations that generate the greatest value for patients will eventually win out. To paraphrase Robert Brook, MCOs are not the problem; poor information and anticompetitive behavior are.

Admittedly, the barriers to improving information and assuring competition are formidable, and if any barriers remain unbroken, the managed care solution may fail. The federal government will have to take a lead role in facilitating coordinated data collection. To assure competition, the courts will have to recognize that powerful providers and powerful MCOs are not the best agents for patients. More important, patients and physicians must be active drivers of competition. It is not enough for patients to complain about quality. They must be willing to withdraw their business from low-quality providers and protest to employers who offer low-quality MCOs. High-quality MCOs and providers can help make this happen by acknowledging that quality varies and by working to improve quality measurement. If these obstacles are overcome, the prerequisites for an efficient market-based health economy will have been met. Physicians will work with MCOs to help patients solve the shopping problem. The evolution from Marcus Welby to managed care will be complete.

Notes

Chapter 1

1. Marcus Welby was not the first icon of trustworthiness. In 1976, President Richard Lyman of Stanford University wrote, ". . . We yearn for the time when good old Jean Hersholt, Hollywood's favorite MD, went around with his battered old black bag curing the sick and comforting the worried." Richard Lyman, "Public Rights and Private Responsibilities: A University Viewpoint," *Journal of Medical Education* 51 (1976): 9. Jean Hersholt appeared as a physician in movies as far back as the 1920s.

2. Harris Co. release, April 27, 1999.

3. K. Arrow, "Uncertainty and the Welfare Economics of Medical Care," *American Economic Review* 53 (1963): 941–73.

4. For example, Regina Hertzlinger, *Market-Driven Health Care* (Reading, Mass.: Addison-Wesley, 1997) and Michael Millenson, *Demanding Medical Excellence* (Chicago: University of Chicago Press, 1997) have written books envisioning a major role for patients in medical decision making.

5. This includes new drugs and new applications of existing drugs.

6. J. Coleman, *Foundations of Social Theory* (Cambridge, Mass.: Harvard University Press, 1990), 91; emphasis added.

7. David Mechanic has written extensively on the evolution of trust in American medicine. A good reference is D. Mechanic, "The Functions and Limitations of Trust in the Provision of Medical Care," *Journal of Health Politics, Policy, and Law*, 23 (1998): 661–86.

8. Ibid., 667

9. Insulin, which was developed in the 1920s, offered the first real treatment for disease. Surgical mortality rates remained unacceptably high until the discovery of antibiotics in the late 1940s.

10. Physicians tend to have higher annual incomes, but they must first endure eight to ten years of medical school and residency training. From the perspective of a college senior, the discounted net present value of the physician's earnings is comparable to that of other professionals' earnings.

11. Mechanic, "The Functions and Limitations of Trust," 667.

12. R. Brook, "Managed Care Is Not the Problem, Quality Is," *Journal of the American Medical Association* 278 (1998): 1612–14.

13. Quoted in D. Enos, and P. Sultan, *The Sociology of Health Care: Social, Economic and Political Perspectives* (New York: Praeger, 1977), p. 64.

14. Ibid. This theme runs throughout their book.

15. V. Fuchs, *Who Shall Live?* (New York: Basic Books, 1974), 56.

16. Ibid., 57.

17. M. Pauly, *Doctors and Their Workshops* (Chicago: University of Chicago Press, 1980).

18. Mechanic, "The Functions and Limitations of Trust."

19. J. Harris, "The Internal Organization of Hospitals: Some Economic Implications," *Bell Journal of Economics* (1977): 8, 473–74; emphasis added.

20. K. Arrow, "Uncertainty and the Welfare Economics of Medical Care," 208.

21. M. A. Morrisey, G. J. Wedig, and M. Hassan, "Do Non-profit Hospitals Pay Their Way?" *Health Affairs* 15, no. 4 (1996): 132–44.

22. M. Friedman, "The Social Responsibility of Business Is to Increase Its Profits," *New York Times Magazine*, September 13, 1970.

23. The arguments offered here were first made by Harry Hansman and then developed more fully by Burton Weisbrod. See H. Hansman, "The Role of Nonprofit Enterprise," *Yale Law Review* 89 (1980): 835–99; and B. Weisbrod, *The Nonprofit Economy* (Cambridge, Mass.: Harvard University Press, 1988).

24. Most nonprofits, including virtually all nonprofit hospitals, are considered charitable organizations. They receive special tax status but in return must provide charitable services and may not base compensation on profits. Other nonprofits, including many nonprofit insurers, are not charitable, do not receive the same tax treatment, and may base compensation on profits.

25. Admittedly, this is just a conjecture. There is no study to date documenting such a micro-level difference between nonprofits and for-profits. This particular issue will soon be moot because a new rule requires the use of safety catheters.

26. The first of a series of articles to make this suggestion is J. Newhouse, "Toward a Theory of Nonprofit Institutions: An Economic Model of a Hospital," *American Economic Review* 60 (1970): 64–74.

27. M. Pauly, M. and M. Redisch, "The Not-for-Profit Hospital as a Physicians' Cooperative," *American Economic Review* 63 (1973): 87–99.

28. W. Miller, Letter, *Hospitals*, July 1, 1967.

29. There were some exceptions. Regulations in a few states permitted insurers to pay fixed fees per admission or per diem. In a few other states, hospitals agreed to an annual budget. These programs were collectively known as *rate setting*. Altogether, there were no more than eight rate-setting states.

30. There have been many studies of cost-shifting by nonprofits, including D. Dranove, "Pricing by Nonprofit Institutions: The Case of Hospital Cost-Shifting," *Journal of Health Economics* 7 (1988): 47–57.

31. See M. Morrisey, *Cost-Shifting in Healthcare: Separating Evidence from Rhetoric* (Washington, D.C.: American Enterprise Institute Press, 1994); and D. Dranove and W. D. White, "Medicaid-Dependent Hospitals and Their Patients: How Have They Fared?" *Health Services Research* 33 (1998): 163–85.

32. J. Gruber, "The Effect of Price Shopping in Medical Markets: Hospital Responses to PPOs in California" (National Bureau of Economic Research, working paper 4190, 1992).

33. B. Gray, *For-Profit Enterprise in Health Care* (Washington, D.C.: National Academy Press, 1986), 187.

34. Weisbrod, *The Nonprofit Economy*.

35. F. Sloan et al., "Hospital Ownership and Cost and Quality of Care: Is There a Dime's Worth of Difference?" (National Bureau of Economic Research, working paper 6706, 1998).

36. D. Himmelstein et al., "Quality of Care in Investor-Owned vs. Not-for-Profit HMOs," *Journal of the American Medical Association* 282 (1999): 159–63.

Chapter 2

1. Insurers may require patients to pay *coinsurance*, which is a fixed percentage of the medical bill, or a *deductible*, which is an up-front fee prior to the beginning of coverage.

2. Anne Scitovsky and Nelda McCall resolved the problem of selection bias by studying a "quasi-experiment" in which Stanford University imposed a 25 percent copayment for physician services. See A. Scitovsky and N. McCall, "Coinsurance and the Demand for Physician Services: Four Years Later," *Social Security Bulletin* 35, no. 6 (1977): 3–19. Using a before-and-after comparison (in which the health status of the Stanford employees presumably did not change very much), they found that the imposition of the copayment led to a 24 percent reduction in physician visits.

3. For a good summary of the RAND study and its findings, see C. Phelps, *Health Economics* (Reading, Mass.: Addison-Wesley, 1997).

4. Arrow, "Uncertainty and the Welfare Economics of Medical Care" 188.

5. P. Starr, *The Social Transformation of American Medicine* (New York: Basic Books, 1982), 6.

6. A natural experiment is a natural event that can be studied as if it were an experiment; that is, without concern for bias. See M. Roemer, "Bed Supply and Hospital Utilization: A Natural Experiment," *Hospitals* 35: (1961): 36–42.

7. Roemer's "test" for inducement is hardly compelling. If physicians could induce demand, why was the hospital occupancy rate so low prior to the expansion?

8. V. Fuchs, "The Supply of Surgeons and the Demand for Operations," *Journal of Human Resources* 13, suppl.: (1978): 35–56.

9. Researchers have attempted to resolve causality using sophisticated statistical techniques, but these efforts have been largely unsuccessful. See J. Ramsey, "A Re-evaluation of Supply and Demand Concepts in Physician Care," report submitted to the Department of Health and Human Services, contract No. HRA 79-0068; and C. Phelps, "Induced Demand: Can We Ever Know Its Extent?" *Journal of Health Economics* 5 (1986): 355–65, for critiques of these methods.

10. Examples of such studies include Office of Inspector General, *Financial Arrangements between Physicians and Health Care Businesses* (Washington, D.C.: Department of Health and Human Services, 1989): B. Hillman et al., "Physicians' Utilization and Charges for Outpatient Diagnostic Imaging in a Medicare Population," *Journal of the American Medical Association* 268 (1992): 2050–54; and B. Hillman, et al., "Frequency and Cost of Diagnostic Imaging in Office Practices: A Comparison of Self-Referring and Radiology-Referring Physicians," *New England Journal of Medicine* 323 (1990): 1604–5.

11. J. Gruber and M. Owings, "Physician Financial Incentives and Cesarean Section Delivery," *RAND Journal of Economics* 27 (1996): 99–123.

12. W. Yip, "Physician Response to Medicare Fee Reductions: Changes in the Volume of Coronary Artery Bypass Graft Surgeries in the Medicare and Private Sectors," *Journal of Health Economics* 17 (1998): 675–700.

13. It is possible that some of the increase is a demand response. When prices fall, patient copayments fall as well, which might drive up demand. But it seems unlikely that patients would be so price sensitive without encouragement from their physicians.

14. J. Gruber, J. Kim, and D. Mayzlin, "Physician Fees and Procedure Intensity: The Case of Cesarean Delivery" (National Bureau of Economic Research, working paper 6744, 1998).

15. The RAND findings would support Enthoven's view. Fully insured patients consumed 30 percent more medical care services than did patients making copayments, yet they had similar health status.

16. This information is drawn from T. Mayer and G. Mayer, "HMOs: Origins and Development," *New England Journal of Medicine* 312 (1985): 590–94.

17. Starr, *The Social Transformation of American Medicine*.

18. Ibid., 216.

19. C. Cutting, "Historical Development and Operating Concepts," in *The Kaiser-Permanente Medical Program*, ed. A. Somers (New York: Commonwealth Fund, 1971).

20. G. Williams, *Kaiser-Permanente Health Plan: Why It Works* (Oakland, Calif.: Kaiser Foundation, 1991).

21. HMOs have no greater incentive to keep their patients healthy than do standard indemnity plans. Both prosper when medical costs are low.

22. W. Crowley, *To Serve the Greatest Number: A History of the Group Health Cooperative of Puget Sound* (Seattle: University of Washington Press, 1996).

23. Cutting, "Historical Development and Operating Concepts," 20.

24. S. Shortell, *A Model of Physician Referral Behavior: A Test of Exchange Theory in Medical Practice*, University of Chicago Center for Health Administration Studies Research Series No. 31. On a related theme, economists Scott Stern and Manuel Trajtenberg recently found that many physicians do a poor job of matching prescription drugs to their patients' specific medical needs. In a sense, they use a narrow "referral" network of drugs, rather than prescribe what is in each patient's best interests. S. Stern and M. Trajtenberg, "Empirical Implications of Physician Authority in Pharmaceutical Decision Making" (National Bureau of Economic Research, working paper 6851, 1998).

25. J. Pulido, A. Hartz, and E. Kuhn, "Are the Best Coronary Artery Bypass Surgeons Identified by Physician Surveys?" *American Journal of Public Health* 87 (1997): 1645–48.

26. P. Franks, et al., "Variations in Primary Care Physicians, Referral Rates," *Health Services Research* 34, no. 1 (1999): 323–29.

27. Williams, *Kaiser-Permanente Health Plan*, 17.

28. Ibid.

29. H. Luft, "How Do Health Maintenance Organizations Achieve Their 'Savings'?" *New England Journal of Medicine* 298 (1978): 1336–43.

30. Ibid.

31. W. Manning et al. "A Controlled Trial of the Effect of a Prepaid Group Practice on the Use of Services." *New England Journal of Medicine* 310 (1984): 1505–10.

Chapter 3

1. See A. Somers, and H. Somers, *Health and Health Care: Policies in Perspective* (Germantown, Md.: Aspen, 1977), for a discussion of the classic arguments against a market-driven health economy. Somers and Somers were not alone in forecasting the inevitable emergence of a tightly regulated national health system.

2. B. Weisbrod, "The Health Care Quadrilemma: An Essay on Technological Change, Insurance, Quality of Care, and Cost Containment," *Journal of Economic Literature* 29 (1991): 523–52.

3. Quoted in C. Adams, "Medical Arms Race: Excess Technology Adds to Soaring Cost," *Times Picayune*, October 16, 1984, A13.

4. J. Robinson and H. Luft, "The Impact of Hospital Market Structure on Patient Volume, Average Length of Stay, and the Cost of Care," *Journal of Health Economics* 4 (1985): 333–56.

5. For a review of this literature, see H. Luft et al., *Hospital Volume, Physician Volume, and Patient Outcomes: Assessing the Evidence*, Health Administration Press Perspectives (Ann Arbor, Mich.: Health Administration Press, 1990).

6. This relationship may also reflect referral patterns, whereby patients are referred to hospitals that have better outcomes.

7. There have been no studies of this possible adverse outcome.

8. See R. Stevens, *Welfare Medicine in America* (New York: Free Press, 1994), for an excellent discussion of the legislative history of the Kerr-Mills, Medicaid, and Medicare programs.

9. These were Connecticut, Maryland, Massachusetts, New Jersey, Rhode Island, Washington, and Wisconsin.

10. Perhaps the seminal study is F. Sloan, "Rate Regulation as a Strategy for Hospital Cost Control," *Milbank Memorial Fund Quarterly* 61 (1983): 195–221. More recent studies found rate setting to be less effective. For example, see J. Antel, R. L. Ohsfeldt, and E. Becker, "State Regulation and Hospital Cost Performance," *REStat* 77 (1995): 416–22.

11. D. Dranove and K. Cone, "Do State Rate Setting Laws Really Lower Hospital Expenses?" *Journal of Health Economics* 4 (1985): 159–65. This difference persists even after controlling for demographic changes and other potential statistical causes.

12. M. Morrisey, F. Sloan, and J. Valvona, "Medicare Prospective Payment and Post-hospital Transfers," *Medical Care* 26 (1988): 685–98.

13. E. Sussman and K. Langa, "The Effect of Cost-Containment Policies on Rates of Coronary Revascularization in California," *New England Journal of Medicine* 329 (1993): 1784–89.

14. D. Dranove and W. White, "Medicaid-Dependent Hospitals and Their Patients: How Have They Fared? *Health Services Research* 33 (1998): 163–85.

15. A. Schwartz, D. Colby, and A. Reisinger, "Variation in Medicaid Physician Fees," *Health Affairs* 10 (spring 1991): 131–39.

16. The difference cannot be explained by the fact that Medicare patients are elderly and tend to be sicker, unless they have become relatively more sick between 1985 and 1997.

17. With the impending revolution in medical care associated with the discovery of the entire human genome, such forecasts must surely be offered with great caution.

18. L. Coggeshall, *Planning for Medical Progress through Education* (Washington, D.C.: Association of American Medical Colleges, 1965), 26.

19. "Summary Report of the Graduate Medical Education National Advisory Council to the Secretary, Department of Health and Human Services," DHHS Publication no. (HRA) 81–651 (Washington, D.C.: U.S. Department of Health and Human Services, 1980).

20. M. Noether, "The Effect of Government Policy Changes on the Supply of Physicians: Expansion of a Competitive Fringe," *Journal of Law and Economics* 29 (1986): 231–62.

21. S. Williams and P. Torrens (*Introduction to Health Services* [New York: Wiley, 1988] detail the history of federal facilities planning legislation.

22. "The Philadelphia Medical Commons: The Choices Ahead," in *Health and Health Care*, ed. A. Somers and H. Somers (Germantown, Md.: Aspen, 1977), 251.

23. The most widely cited study is D. Salkever and T. Bice, "The Impact of Certificate of Need Controls on Hospital Investment," *Milbank Quarterly* 54 (1976): 185–214.

24. M. Morrisey, "State Health Care Reform: Protecting the Provider," in *American Health Care: Government, Market Processes, and the Public Interest*, ed. M. Morrisey (Oakland, Cailf.: The Independent Institute, 1999).

25. C. Conover and F. Sloan, "Does Removing Certificate-of-Need Regulations Lead to a Surge in Health Care Spending?" *Journal of Health Politics, Policy, and Law* 23 (1998): 455–81.

26. C. Simon, D. Dranove, and W. White, "The Impact of Managed Care on the Physician Marketplace," *Public Health Reports* 112 (1977): 222–30.

27. J. Moore, "Med School Applicants Drop Again," *Modern Healthcare*, September 12, 1999.

28. The program also covered patients in a separate Maternal and Child Health program.

29. A community hospital can be for-profit, nonprofit, or owned by a state or local government agency. It provides general medical services for inpatients with short lengths of stay (averaging thirty days or less).

30. Quoted in B. Mittler, "The Demise of the SuperMeds," *Best's Review—Life Insurance Edition* 87 (1987): 50.

31. "Prescription for Profits: Private Hospital Firms Bring Management Skills to the Bedside," *Time*, July 4, 1983, 42.

32. A. Relman, "The New Medical-Industrial Complex," *New England Journal of Medicine* 303 (1980): 963. This expression is a reworking of the phrase "the military-industrial complex," coined by President Eisenhower to warn Americans about the dangers of such an alliance.

33. D. Mechanic, "Changing Medical Organization and the Erosion of Trust," *Millbank Quarterly* 74 (1996): 171–89.

34. For example, see R. Pattison and H. Katz, "Investor-Owned and Not-for-Profit Hospitals: A Comparison Based on California Data," *New England Journal of Medicine* 309 (1982): 347–53; F. Sloan and R. Vraciu, "Investor-Owned and Not-for-Profit Hospitals: Addressing Some Issues," *Health Affairs* 2 (spring 1983): 25–34; J. Watt et al., "The Comparative Economic Performance of Investor-Owned Chain and Not-for-Profit Hospitals," *New England Journal of Medicine* 314 (1986): 89–96.

35. This does not include indirect costs of Medicare, such as distortions in labor markets created by the Medicare payroll tax.

36. Medicare is administered within each state by private health insurers—the same insurers who offer indemnity and managed care products to the under-sixty-five population. The difference in administrative costs between Medicare and private insurance is the direct result of marketing and medical underwriting.

Chapter 4

1. U.S. Council on Wage and Price Stability, cited in L. Brown, "Dogmatic Slumbers," in *The Politics of Health Care Reform*, ed. James Marone and Gary Belkin (Durham, N.C.: Duke University Press, 1994).

2. J. Cantor et al., "Data Watch: Business Leaders' Views on American Health Care," *Health Affairs* 10 (1991): 98–105.

3. Most notably, A. Enthoven, "Consumer-Choice Health Plan: Inflation and Inequity in Health Care Today: Alternatives for Cost Control and an Analysis of Proposals for National Health Insurance," *New England Journal of Medicine* 298 (1978): 650–659, 709–19.

4. A. Enthoven, and R. Kronick, "A Consumer-Choice Health Plan for the 1990s," *New England Journal of Medicine* 320 (1989) 29–37.

5. Quoted in I. Miller, *American Health Care Blues* (New Brunswick, N.J.: Transaction, 1996).

6. H. E. Frech, "Preferred Provider Organizations and Health Care Competition," in *Health Care in America*, ed. H. E. Frech (San Francisco: Pacific Research Institute for Public Policy, 1988), 353–70.

7. Employers self-insure by paying for their employee's medical bills on an ongoing basis rather than pay premiums to an insurance company. In this way, employers continue to bear the financial risk for the medical expenditures of their employees. Many firms, including benefits management companies and insurers, help companies establish self-insured plans.

8. These widely different estimates reflect differences in defining PPOs and in the survey methods used to identify PPO enrollment.

9. For a summary of several studies, see Center for Health Policy Research, *Economic Impacts of Managed Care Reform* (Chicago: American Medical Association, 1999).

10. To avoid state legislation, many employers will simply offer their own MCOs. But employers will be unable to avoid the cost increases that will result from a federal "patient bill of rights."

11. D. Dranove, M. Shanley, and W. White, "Price and Concentration in Hospital Markets: The Shift from Patient-Driven to Payer-Driven Competition," *Journal of Law and Economics* 36 (1993): 179–204.

12. There is abundant evidence that hospitals set lower prices in the face of competition. See D. Dranove, and M. Satterthwaite, "The Industrial Organization of Health Care," and M. Gaynor, "Antitrust," both in *The Handbook of Health Economics*, ed. J. Newhouse, forthcoming.

13. Times change. My Cornell professors characterized 1970s HMOs as offering Volkswagen treatment instead of Cadillac treatment.

14. C. Pantilat, M. Chesney, and B. Lo, "Effect of Incentives on the Use of Indicated Services in Managed Care" *Western Journal of Medicine* 170 (1999): 137–42.

15. A. Hillman, M. Pauly, and J. Kerstein, "How Do Financial Incentives Affect Physicians' Clinical Decisions and the Financial Performance of Health Maintenance Organizations?" *New England Journal of Medicine* 321 (1989): 86–92.

16. G. Hickson, W. Altmeier, and J. Perrin, "Physician Reimbursement by Salary or Fee-for-Service: Effect on Physician Practice Behavior in a Randomized Prospective Study" *Pediatrics* 80 (1987): 344–50.

17. It is sometimes possible to use sophisticated statistical techniques to avoid selection bias. But the data requirements are severe and do not appear to have been fully met by existing studies.

18. In *Health Economics*, Charles Phelps reports that the first study of practice variations appeared in 1938. That study of British school children found a tenfold difference in the rate of tonsillectomies across regions of the country.

19. J. Wennberg, J. Freeman, and W. Culp, "Are Hospital Services Rationed in New Haven or Over-utilised in Boston?" *Lancet* 1 (1987): 1185–88. Note that Boston has much greater hospital capacity. Phelps and Mooney observe that the fact that Boston residents are not systematically overtreated is a direct refutation of Roemer's law.

20. *Dartmouth Atlas of Health Care*, ed. Jack Wennberg (Chicago: American Hospital Publishing, 1996, 1999).

21. G. O'Conner et al., "Geographic Variation in the Treatment of Acute Myocardial Infarction: The Cooperative Cardiovascular Project," *Journal of the American Medical Association* 281 (1999): 627–33.

22. For novice statisticians, roughly one-third of a set of values lies at least one standard deviation above or below the mean value.

23. Phelps, *Health Economics*.

24. C. Phelps and C. Mooney, "Variations in Medical Practice Use: Causes and Consequences," in *Competitive Approaches to Health Care Reform*, ed. D. Arnould, R. Rich, and W. White (Washington, D.C.: Urban Institute Press, 1993).

25. C. Phelps, et al., "Doctors Have Styles—and They Matter!" (University of Rochester working paper, 1994).

26. Phelps, *Health Economics*.

27. Quoted in R. Winslow, "Elderly Need Preventive Care but Don't Get It," *Wall Street Journal*, April 19, 1999, sec. II, p. B4.

28. Quoted in R. Winslow, "Heart Attack Therapy Varies Sharply by Region," *Wall Street Journal*, February 17, 1999, B5.

29. V. G. Freeman et al., "Lying for Patients: Physician Deception of Third-Party Payers," *Archives of Internal Medicine* (1999): 2263–70; M. Wynia, D. Cummins, and J. VanGeest, "Physician Responses to Utilization Review Pressures: Results of a National Survey" (Chicago: AMA Institute for Ethics, 1999).

30. Quoted in R. Rosenblatt and A. Rubin, "Lag in Health Tests for Medicare Patients Found," *Buffalo News*, April 19, 1999, 4A.

31. T. Wickizer, J. Wheeler, and P. Feldstein, "Does Utilization Review Reduce Unnecessary Hospital Care and Contain Costs?" *Medical Care* 27 (1989): 632–47.

32. T. Wickizer, and D. Lessler, "Do Treatment Restrictions Imposed by Utilization Management Increase the Likelihood of Readmission for Psychiatric Patients?" *Medical Care* 36 (1998): 844–50.

33. Comparisons of expenses as a fraction of GDP are always tricky because they can be affected by changes in the GDP. One important reason that the fraction fell in the mid-1990s was the growth in the GDP, just as one reason the fraction increased in the early 1990s was the recession. Even so, the most important reason for the decline is the slowdown in the rate of growth of health care expenditures, especially for privately insured patients.

34. R. Miller and H. Luft, "Managed Care Plan Performance since 1980: A Literature Analysis," *Journal of the American Medical Association* 271 (1994): 1512–17.

35. D. Cutler, and L. Sheiner, "Managed Care and the Growth of Medical Expenditures" (mimeo, Harvard University, 1997).

36. D. Cutler, M. McClellan, and J. Newhouse, "Prices and Productivity in Managed Care," RAND Journal of Economics, forthcoming.

37. A. Flood et al., "How Do HMOs Achieve Savings?" *Health Services Research* 33 (1998): 79–100.

38. Cutler and Sheiner, "Managed Care and the Growth of Medical Expenditures."

39. D. Cutler, and M. McClellan, "The Determinants of Technological Change in Heart Attack Treatment" (National Bureau of Economic Research, working paper 5751, 1996); M. Chernew, A. M. Fendrick, and R. Hirth, "Managed Care and Medical Technology: Implications for Cost Growth" *Health Affairs* 16 (1997): 196–206.

40. S. Hill, and B. Wolfe, "Testing the HMO Competitive Strategy," *Journal of Health Economics* 16 (1997): 261–86.

41. For example, in a 1997 ABC News survey, 88 percent of HMO enrollees reported that they were satisfied with the quality of care, compared with 92 percent of enrollees in traditional plans. The difference of 4 percent was not statistically meaningful.

42. F. Hellinger, "The Impact of Managed Care on Market Performance: A Review of New Evidence" (mimeo, Agency for Health Care Policy and Research, 1996).

43. R. Miller and H. Luft, "Managed Care Performance: Is Quality of Care Better or Worse?" *Health Affairs* 16, no. 5 (1997): 7–25.

44. J. Seidman et al., "Review of Studies That Compare the Quality of Cardiovascular Care in HMO versus Non-HMO Settings," *Medical Care* 36 (1998): 1607–25.

45. T. Soumerai et al., "Timeliness and Quality of Care for Elderly Patients with Acute Myocardial Infarction under Health Maintenance Organizations vs. Fee-for-Service Insurance," *Archives of Internal Medicine* 159 (1999): 2013–20.

46. G. Riley et al., "Stage at Diagnosis and Treatment Patterns among Older Women with Breast Cancer: An HMO and Fee-for-Service Comparison," *Journal of the American Medical Association* 281 (1999): 720–26; Schnelle et al., "Objective and Subjective Measures of the Quality of Managed Care in Nursing Homes," *Medical Care* 37 (1999): 375–83.

47. J. Ware et al., "Differences in 4-Year Health Outcomes for Elderly and Poor, Chronically Ill Patients Treated in HMO and Fee-for-Service Systems," *Journal of the American Medical Association* 276 (1996): 1039–47.

48. Henry Kaiser Family Foundation/Harvard University/Princeton Survey Research Associates Poll (Storrs, Conn.: Roper Center for Public Opinion Research, August 22, 1997).

49. See A. Kao et al., "The Relationship between Method of Physician Payment and Patient Trust," *Journal of the American Medical Association* 280 (1998): 1708–14.

50. See K. Grumbach et al., "Resolving the Gatekeeper Condundrum," *Journal of the American Medical Association* 282 (1999): 261–66.

Chapter 5

1. Both tax rules and insurer preferences for dealing with large groups favor employer purchase of health insurance over individual purchases.

2. *Management Strategies Used by Large Employers to Control Costs*, U.S. General Accounting Office Report 97–71 (Washington, D.C.: U.S. General Accounting Office, 1997).

3. See P. Cunningham et al., "Managed Care and Physicians' Provision of Charity Care," *Journal of the American Medical Association* 281 (1999): 1087–92, and J. Weissman et al., "Market Forces and Unsponsored Research in Academic Health Centers," *Journal of the American Medical Association* 281 (1999): 1093–98.

4. See M. Ullman et al., "Performance Measurement in Prostate Cancer Care: Beyond Report Cards," *Urology* 47 (1996): 356–65.

5. S. Shortell et al., "Assessing the Impact of Continuous Quality Improvement on Clinical Practice: What It Will Take to Accelerate Progress," *Milbank Quarterly* 76 (1998): 593–625.

6. Steering Committee on Clinical Practice Guidelines for the Care and Treatment of Breast Cancer, "Adjuvant Systematic Therapy for Women with Node-Positive Breast Cancer," *Canadian Medical Association Journal* 158, S3 (1998): S52–S64.

7. K. Sandrick, "Out in Front: Managed Care Helps Push Clinical Guidelines Forward," *Hospitals* 67, no. 9 (1993): 30–31.

8. Quoted in D. Moskowitz, "Coloradians Tame the Guidelines Beast," *Business and Health* 16, no. 10 (1998): 63–64.

9. Quoted in Sandrick, "Out in Front."

10. AHCPR often uses the term *guidelines* to describe what I call disease management.

11. M. Fine et al., "The Hospital Admission Decision for Patients with Community-Acquired Pneumonia: Results from the Pneumonia Patient Outcomes Research Team," *Archives of Internal Medicine* 157 (1997): 36–44.

12. J. Sisk, "How Are Health Care Organizations Using Clinical Guidelines?" *Health Affairs* 17, no. 5 (1998): 91–109.

13. See Moskowitz, "Coloradians Tame the Guidelines Beast," 63–64.

14. M. Dean, "A Quiet Clinical Guideline Revolution Begins," *Lancet* 353 (1999): 650.

15. I have had the opportunity to examine the structure of managed care networks both in a number of antitrust cases and in conjunction with executive education programs. It is remarkable how certain basic patterns—"hub" teaching hospital and wide geographic access—are present throughout the nation. Some employers even specify these requirements when contracting with MCOs.

16. Jack Zwanziger and Adam Meirowitz find, however, that teaching hospitals are less likely to be included in a managed care network. In other words, managed care plans want one teaching hospital in their network, but they may not want a second. See J. Zwanziger and A. Meirowitz, "Strategic Factors in Hospital Selection for HMO and PPO Networks," in *Managed Care and Changing Health Care Markets*, ed. M. Morrisey (Washington, D.C.: American Enterprise Institute, 1998).

17. This and all the other comparisons in this section hold true even if we control for specialty.

18. The expense of $500 generates a total QALY gain of 0.4 QALYs. Hence, the cost per QALY is $500/.4 = $1,250.

19. The expense of $200 generates a total QALY gain of 0.25 QALYs. Hence, the cost per QALY is $200/.25 = $800.

20. A. Laupacis et al., 1992 "How Attractive Does a New Technology Have to Be to Warrant Adoption and Utilization?" *Canadian Medical Journal* 146 (1992): 473–81.

21. J. D. Kleinke, "Release 0.0: Clinical Information Technology in the Real World," *Health Affairs* 17, no. 6 (1998): 23–38.

22. Ibid., 29.

23. For example, Thomas Buchmueller and Paul Feldstein found that 25 percent of University of California employees enrolled in MCOs would switch plans to save $100 annually. See T. Buchmueller and P. Feldstein, "The Effect of Price on Switching among Health Plans," *Journal of Health Economics*, 16 (1997): 231–48.

Chapter 6

1. Altogether, BJC owns fourteen hospitals, as well as six nursing homes. It also offers its own health plan.

2. For a good discussion of the pitfalls of mergers, see M. Sirower, *The Synergy Trap* (New York: Free Press, 1997).

3. Fixed costs are costs that must be incurred whether a firm produces one or one million units.

4. W. Lynk, "The Creation of Economic Efficiencies in Hospital Mergers," *Journal of Health Economics* 14 (1995): 507–30.

5. Hill, and Wolfe, "Testing the HMO Competitive Strategy."

6. Quoted in M. Blechner, "Size Does Matter," *Hospitals and Health Networks*, June 20, 1998, 30.

7. D. Dranove, "Economies of Scale in Non-Revenue-Producing Cost Centers in Hospitals," *Journal of Health Economics* 7 (1988): 47–57.

8. A paper that does a good job of explaining the statistical issues is M. Long, "A Reconsideration of Economies of Scale in the Health Care Field," *Health Policy* 5 (1985): 25–44.

9. J. Greene, "Do Mergers Work?" *Modern Healthcare*, March 19, 1990, 24; and J. Greene, "The Costs of Hospital Mergers" *Modern Healthcare*, February 3, 1992, 36.

10. G. Colon, A, Gupta, and P. Mango, "M&A Malpractice," *McKinsey Quarterly*, no. 1 (1999): 62–77.

11. D. Dranove, A. Durkac, and M. Shanley, "Are Multihospital Systems More Efficient?" *Health Affairs* 15, no. 1 (1996): 100–104.

12. R. Conner, R. Feldman, and B. Dowd, "The Effects of Market Concentration and Horizontal Mergers on Hospital Costs and Prices" (Mimeo, University of Minnesota, 1997).

13. M. Guo, "Incentives and Effects of Hospital Mergers under Managed Care: Theory and Evidence" (Ph.D. dissertation, Northwestern University, 1999).

14. R. Given, "Economies of Scale and Scope as an Explanation of Merger and Output Diversification Activities in the Health Maintenance Organization Industry," *Journal of Health Economics* 15 (1996): 685–714.

15. Federal antikickback statutes and ethical codes prevent hospitals from paying for referrals, necessitating the acquisition.

16. See Dranove and Satterthwaite, "The Industrial Organization of Health Care," for a review of the evidence. This turns out to be somewhat tricky to show. One problem comes from trying to make apples-to-apples comparisons of prices across different providers who may be offering slightly different services or treating patients with different severities of illness. Another problem arises from difficulties in obtaining the actual prices paid by MCOs.

17. The plaintiff in the case was another radiologist who complained that the monopoly group prevented his practicing in the town. The court ultimately found for the defense, arguing that regardless of whether the group was a monopoly, it did not illegally block entry by the plaintiff.

18. There are no rules specifying which agency will file the challenge. In general, the DOJ tends to tackle higher profile antitrust cases, but there are exceptions.

19. Several researchers have documented the bargaining power of large purchasers. For example, see G. Melnick et al., "The Effects of Market Structure and Bargaining Position on Hospital Prices," *Journal of Health Economics* 11 (1992): 217–33.

20. See F. Scott-Morton, "The Strategic Response by Pharmaceutical Firms to

the Medicaid Most-Favored-Customer Rules," *RAND Journal of Economics* 28, (1997): 269–90.

21. For evidence on physician locations, see C. Simon, D. Dranove, and W. White, "The Impact of Managed Care on the Physician Marketplace," *Public Health Reports* 112 (1997): 222–30.

22. It is difficult to get good data on this. My colleague Martin Gaynor reports that in just one year, 1994–95, the number of physician practices owned by hospitals increased from 7,015 to 11,234.

23. J. Robinson, "Vertical Integration and Organizational Networks in Health Care," *Health Affairs* 15, no. 1 (1996): 7–22.

Chapter 7

1. Brook, "Managed Care Is Not the Problem, Quality Is," 1612–14.

2. Stern and Trajtenberg, "Empirical Implications of Physician Authority in Pharmaceutical Decision Making."

3. Harold Luft does a good job reviewing this and related evidence in Luft et al., *Hospital Volume, Physician Volume, and Patient Outcomes*.

4. Edward Hannan provides a nice overview of the reasons against relying too much on experience as an indicator of quality. E. Hannan, "The Relation between Volume and Outcome in Health Care," *New England Journal of Medicine* 340 (1999): 1677–79.

5. Cited in the Advisory Board Company, "The Imperative and Opportunity for Disease Management" (Presentation to Merck & Company, May 22, 1999).

6. J. Chen et al., "Do America's Best Hospitals Perform Better for Acute Myocardial Infarction?" *New England Journal of Medicine* 340 (1999): 286–92.

7. Advisory Board Company, *The Imperative and Opportunity for Disease Management*.

8. J. Chen et al., "Performance of the '100 Top Hospitals': What Does the Report Card Mean?" *Health Affairs* 18, no. 4 (1999): 53–68.

9. R. Thaler and S. Rosen, "The Value of Saving a Life: Evidence from the Labor Market," in *Household Production and Consumption*, ed. N. Terlecky (New York: National Bureau of Economic Research, 1975).

10. W. K. Viscusi, "The Value of Risks to Life and Health," *Journal of Economic Literature* 31 (1993): 1912–46.

11. G. Tolley, D. Kenkel, and R. Fabian, *Valuing Health for Policy: An Economic Approach* (Chicago: University of Chicago Press, 1994).

12. D. Cutler and E. Richardson, "Your Money and Your Life: The Value of Health and What Affects It" (National Bureau of Economic Research, working paper 6895, 1999).

13. For more on QALYs, see R. Kaplan, "Utility Assessment for Estimating Quality-Adjusted Life Years," in *Valuing Health Care: Costs, Benefits, and Effectiveness of Pharmaceuticals, and Other Medical Technologies*, ed. F. Sloan (Cambrige: Cambridge University Press, 1995), 31–60.

14. A. Karlan, "Rankings Miss Hospitals' Human Side," *Chicago Tribune*, November 10, 1998, sec. 1, p. 26.

15. A. Donabedian, *Exploration in Quality Assessment and Monitoring*, vol. 1, *The Definition of Quality and Approaches to Its Assessment* (Ann Arbor, Mich.: Health Administration Press, 1980).

16. T. Brennan et al., "Incidence of Adverse Events and Negligence in Hospitalized Patients: Results of the Harvard Medical Practice Study," *New England Journal of Medicine* 324 (1991): 370–74.

17. J. Geraci et al., "The Association of Quality of Care and Occurrence of In-Hospital, Treatment-Related Complications," *Medical Care* 37 (1999): 140–48.

18. E. Schneider and A. Epstein, "Influence of Cardiac-Surgery Performance Reports on Referral Practices and Access to Care: A Survey of Cardiovascular Specialists," *New England Journal of Medicine* 335 (1996): 251–56.

19. Quoted in T. Burton, "Heart-Care Assessment Finds Reputation and Reality Don't Necessarily Match," *Wall Street Journal Interactive Edition*, April 22, 1999.

20. D. Dranove and M. Satterthwaite, "Monopolistic Competition When Price and Quality Are Not Perfectly Observable," *RAND Journal of Economics* 23 (1992): 518–34.

21. We also considered a third dimension of quality: finding the right match between patient and provider. Providers have different styles of practice and experience, and the provider who is best for one patient may not be best for another.

22. Schneider and Epstein, "Influence of Cardiac-Surgery Performance Reports."

23. I am grateful to Mark Satterthwaite for this theoretical insight.

24. J. Ware and C. Sherbourne, "The MOS 36-Item Short-Form Health Survey (SF-36): I. Conceptual Framework and Item Selection," *Medical Care* 30 (1992): 473–83.

25. Some of these organizations use variants of these scales to predict hospital expenditures.

26. S. Mennemeyer, M. Morrisey, and L. Howard, "Death and Reputation: How Consumers Acted upon HCFA Mortality Information," *Inquiry* 34 (1997): 117–28.

27. D. Mukamel and A. Mushlin, "Quality of Care Information Makes a Difference," *Medical Care* 36 (1998): 945–54.

28. Schneider and Epstein, "Influence of Cardiac-Surgery Performance Reports."

29. Major morbidity is based on a MedisGroups concept and is essentially the actual failure or potential for imminent failure of a major organ. A complication is a secondary diagnosis that appears to be caused by the hospitalization.

30. Personal conversation with Mark Pauly.

31. J. Gabel et al., "When Employers Choose Health Plans: Do NCQA Accreditation and HEDIS Data Count?" *The Commonwealth Fund*, September 1998.

32. E. Delong et al., "The Effects of New York's Bypass Surgery Provider Profiling on Access to Care and Patient Outcomes in the Elderly," *Journal of the American College of Cardiology* 32 (1998): 993–99.

33. D. Dranove, et al., "Quality Information Is Good, Except When It's Not" (mimeo, Northwestern University, 1999).

34. M. Lu et al., "Risk Selection and Matching in Performance-Based Contracting" (mimeo, University of Calgary, 1999). Note that Maine's system rewards improvement in health status, not the level of health status. Thus, providers may have greater incentive to treat the most severely ill patients because they afford the largest opportunity for improvement.

35. J. Escarce et al., "Health Maintenance Organizations and Hospital Quality of Care for Coronary Artery Bypass Surgery," *Medical Care Research and Review* 56 (1999): 340–62.

36. JCAHO Web site.

37. See Kao et al., "The Relationship between Method of Physician Payment and Patient Trust," 1708–14.

38. See M. Weinstein, "Managed Care's Other Problem: It's Not What You Think," *New York Times* February 4, 1999, Sec. 4, pp. 1, 4.

39. H. Schauffler, C. Brown, and A. Milstein, "Raising the Bar: The Use of Performance Guarantees by the Pacific Business Group on Health," *Health Affairs* 18, no. 2 (1999): 134–42. Other regional Business Groups on Health are also engaged in developing and using MCO report cards.

40. Gabel et al., "When Employers Choose Health Plans."

Chapter 8

1. Carol Simon, William White, and I have shown in ongoing research that nearly all the recent consolidation among hospitals can be explained by the growth of managed care. D. Dranove, C. Simon, and W. White, "Is Managed Care Increasing Concentration in Healthcare Markets?" (mimeo, 1999).

2. See D. Dranove, C. Simon, and W. White, "Determinants of Managed Care Penetration," *Journal of Health Economics* 17 (1998): 729–46.

3. White House Domestic Policy Council, *Health Security: The President's Report to the American People*, 1993, 62.

4. The Consumer Assessment of Health Plans (CAHPs) is another instrument that is used to monitor consumer experiences with health plans. See P. D. Cleary, "Satisfaction May Not Suffice! A Commentary on 'A Patient's Perspective,'" *International Journal of Technology Assessment in Health Care*, 14 (1998): 35–37.

5. California Healthcare Foundation survey conducted by Princeton Survey Research Associates, November–December 1998.

6. T. Hofer et al., "The Unreliability of Individual Physician 'Report Cards' for Assessing the Costs and Quality of Care for a Chronic Disease," *Journal of the American Medical Association* 281 (1999): 2098–05.

Bibliography

Adams, C. "Medical Arms Race: Excess Technology Adds to Soaring Cost." *Times Picayune*, October 16, 1984, A13.

Advisory Board Company. "The Imperative and Opportunity for Disease Management." Presentation to Merck & Company, May 22, 1999.

Antel, J., R. L. Ohsfeldt, and E. Becker. "State Regulation and Hospital Cost Performance." *REStat* 77 (1995): 416–22.

Arrow, K. "Agency and the Welfare Economics of Medical Care." *American Economic Review* 53 (1993): 941–73.

Blechner, M. "Size Does Matter?" *Hospitals and Health Networks*, June 20, 1998, 30.

Brennan, T., et al. "Incidence of Adverse Events and Negligence in Hospitalized Patients: Results of the Harvard Medical Practice Study." *New England Journal of Medicine* 324 (1991): 370–74.

Brook, R. "Managed Care Is Not the Problem, Quality Is." *Journal of the American Medical Association* 278 (1998): 1612–14.

Brown, L. "Dogmatic Slumbers." In *The Politics of Health Care Reform*, ed. James Marone and Gary Belkin, 205–23. Durham, N.C.: Duke University Press, 1994.

Buchmueller, T., and P. Feldstein. "The Effect of Price on Switching among Health Plans." *Journal of Health Economics* 16 (1997): 231–48.

Burton, T. "Heart-Care Assessment Finds Reputation and Reality Don't Necessarily Match." *Wall Street Journal Interactive Edition*, April 22, 1999.

Cantor, J., et al., "Data Watch: Business Leaders' Views on American Health Care." *Health Affairs* 10 (1991): 98–105.

Center for Health Policy Research. *Economic Impacts of Managed Care Reform*. Chicago: American Medical Association, 1999.

Chen, J., et al. "Do America's Best Hospitals Perform Better for Acute Myocardial Infarction?" *New England Journal of Medicine* 340 (1999): 286–92.

Chen, J., et al. "Performance of the '100 Top Hospitals': What Does the Report Card Mean?" *Health Affairs* 18, no. 4 (1999): 53–68.

Chernew, M., A. M. Fendrick, and R. Hirth. "Managed Care and Medical Technology: Implications for Cost Growth." *Health Affairs* 16 (1997): 196–206.

Cleary, P. D. "Satisfaction May Not Suffice! A Commentary on 'A Patient's Perspective.'" *International Journal of Technology Assessment in Health Care*, 14, no. 1 (1998): 35–37

Coggeshall, L. *Planning for Medical Progress through Education*. Washington, D.C.: Association of American Medical Colleges, 1965.

Coleman, J. *Foundations of Social Theory*. Cambridge, Mass.: Harvard University Press, 1990.

Collins, T. "In Search of Evidence: California System Adopts Clinical Guidelines, Finds Quality Approach Is Cost-Effective." *Modern Healthcare*, November 9, 1998, 108.

Colon, G., A. Gupta, and P. Mango. "M&A Malpractice." *McKinsey Quarterly*, no. 1 (1999): 62–77.

Conner, R., R. Feldman, and B. Dowd. "The Effects of Market Concentration and Horizontal Mergers on Hospital Costs and Prices." Mimeo, University of Minnesota, 1997.

Conover, C., and F. Sloan. "Does Removing Certificate-of-Need Regulations Lead to a Surge in Health Care Spending?" *Journal of Health Politics, Policy, and Law* 23 (1998): 455–81.

Crowley, W. *To Serve the Greatest Number: A History of the Group Health Cooperative of Puget Sound*. Seattle: University of Washington Press, 1996.

Cunningham, P., et al. "Managed Care and Physicians' Provision of Charity Care." *Journal of the American Medical Association* 281 (1999): 1087–92.

Cutler, D., and M. McClellan. "The Determinants of Technological Change in Heart Attack Treatment." National Bureau of Economic Research, working paper 5751, 1996.

Cutler, D., M. McClellan, and J. Newhouse. "Prices and Productivity in Managed Care." *RAND Journal of Economics*, forthcoming.

Cutler, D., and E. Richardson. "Your Money and Your Life: The Value of Health and What Affects It." National Bureau of Economic Research, working paper 6895, 1999.

Cutler, D., and L. Sheiner. "Managed Care and the Growth of Medical Expenditures." Mimeo, Harvard University, 1997.

Cutting, C. "Historical Development and Operating Concepts." In *The Kaiser-Permanente Medical Program*, ed. A. Somers. New York: Commonwealth Fund, 1971.

Dartmouth Atlas of Health Care. Ed. Jack Wennberg. Chicago: American Hospital Publishing, 1996, 1999.

Dean, M. "A Quiet Clinical Guideline Revolution Begins." *Lancet* 353 (1999): 650.

Delong, E., et al. "The Effects of New York's Bypass Surgery Provider Profiling on Access to Care and Patient Outcomes in the Elderly." *Journal of the American College of Cardiology* 32 (1998): 993–99.

Donabedian, A. *Exploration in Quality Assessment and Monitoring*. Vol. 1, *The Definition of Quality and Approaches to Its Assessment*. Ann Arbor, Mich.: Health Administration Press, 1980.

Dranove, D. "Pricing by Nonprofit Institutions: The Case of Hospital Cost-Shifting." *Journal of Health Economics* 7 (1988): 47–57.

———. "Economies of Scale in Non-Revenue-Producing Cost Centers in Hospitals." *Journal of Health Economics* 17 (1988): 69–83.

Dranove, D., and K. Cone. "Do State Rate Setting Laws Really Lower Hospital Expenses?" *Journal of Health Economics* 4 (1985): 159–65.

Dranove, D., A. Durkac, and M. Shanley. "Are Multihospital Systems More Efficient?" *Health Affairs* 15, no. 1 (1996): 100–104.

Dranove, D., and M. Satterthwaite. "Monopolistic Competition When Price and Quality Are Not Perfectly Observable." *RAND Journal of Economics* 23 (1992): 518–34.

————. "The Industrial Organization of Health Care." In *The Handbook of Health Economics*, ed. J. Newhouse. Forthcoming.

Dranove, D., M. Shanley, and W. White. "Price and Concentration in Hospital Markets: The Shift from Patient-Driven to Payer-Driven Competition." *Journal of Law and Economics* 36 (1993): 179–204.

Dranove, D., C. Simon, and W. White. "Determinants of Managed Care Penetration." *Journal of Health Economics* 17 (1998): 729–46.

————. "Is Managed Care Increasing Concentration in Healthcare Markets?" Mimeo, 1999.

Dranove, D., and W. D. White. "Medicaid-Dependent Hospitals and Their Patients: How Have They Fared?" *Health Services Research* 33 (1998): 163–85.

Dranove, D., et al. "Quality Information Is Good, Except When It's Not." Mimeo, Northwestern University, 1999.

Enos, D., and P. Sultan. *The Sociology of Health Care: Social, Economic and Political Perspectives*. New York: Praeger, 1977.

Enthoven, A. "Consumer-Choice Health Plan. Inflation and Inequity in Health Care Today: Alternatives for Cost Control and an Analysis of Proposals for National Health Insurance." *New England Journal of Medicine* 298 (1978): 650–59, 709–19.

Enthoven, A., and R. Kronick. "A Consumer-Choice Health Plan for the 1990s." *New England Journal of Medicine* 320 (1989): 29–37.

Escarce, J., et al. "Health Maintenance Organizations and Hospital Quality of Care for Coronary Artery Bypass Surgery." *Medical Care Research and Review* 56 (1999): 340–62.

Fine, M., et al. "The Hospital Admission Decision for Patients with Community-Acquired Pneumonia: Results from the Pneumonia Patient Outcomes Research Team." *Archives of Internal Medicine* 157 (1997): 36–44.

Flood, A., et al. "How Do HMOs Achieve Savings?" *Health Services Research* 33 (1998): 79–100.

Franks, P., et al. "Variations in Primary Care Physician's Referral Rates." *Health Services Research* 34 (1999): 323–29.

Frech, H. E. "Preferred Provider Organizations and Health Care Competition." In *Health Care in America*, ed. H. E. Frech. San Francisco: Pacific Research Institute for Public Policy, 1988.

Freeman, V. G., et al. "Lying for Patients: Physician Deception of Third-Party Payers." *Archives of Internal Medicine* (1997): 2263–70.

Friedman, M. "The Social Responsibility of Business Is to Increase Its Profits." *New York Times Magazine*, September 13, 1970.

Fuchs, V. *Who Shall Live?* New York: Basic Books, 1974.

————. "The Supply of Surgeons and the Demand for Operations." *Journal of Human Resources* 13, suppl. (1978): 35–56.

Gabel, J., et al. "When Employers Choose Health Plans: Do NCQA Accreditation and HEDIS Data Count?" *The Commonwealth Fund*, September 1998.

Gaynor, M. "Antitrust." In *The Handbook of Health Economics*, ed. J. Newhouse. Forthcoming.

Geraci, J., et al., "The Association of Quality of Care and Occurrence of In-Hospital, Treatment-Related Complications." *Medical Care* 37 (1999): 140–48.

Given, R. "Economies of Scale and Scope as an Explanation of Merger and Output Diversification Activities in the Health Maintenance Organization Industry." *Journal of Health Economics* 15 (1996): 685–714.

Gray, B. *For-Profit Enterprise in Health Care.* Washington, D.C.: National Academy Press, 1986.

Greene, J. 1990 "Do Mergers Work?" *Modern Healthcare*, March 19, 1990, 24.

———. "The Costs of Hospital Mergers." *Modern Healthcare*, February 3, 1992, 36.

Grimshaw, J., and I. Russell. "Effect of Clinical Guidelines on Medical Practice: A Systematic Review of Rigorous Evaluations." *Lancet* 342 (1993): 1317–22.

Gruber, J. "The Effect of Price Shopping in Medical Markets: Hospital Responses to PPOs in California." National Bureau of Economic Research, working paper 4190, 1992.

Gruber, J., J. Kim, and D. Mayzlin. "Physician Fees and Procedure Intensity: The Case of Cesarean Delivery." National Bureau of Economic Research, working paper 6744, 1998.

Gruber, J., and M. Owings. "Physician Financial Incentives and Cesarean Section Delivery." *RAND Journal of Economics* 27 (1996): 99–123.

Grumbach, K., et al. "Resolving the Gatekeeper Conundrum" *Journal of the American Medical Association* 282 (1999): 261–66.

Guo, M. "Incentives and Effects of Hospital Mergers under Managed Care: Theory and Evidence." Ph.D. dissertation, Northwestern University, 1999.

Hannan, E. "The Relation between Volume and Outcome in Health Care." *New England Journal of Medicine* 340 (1999): 1677–79.

Hansman, H. "The Role of Nonprofit Enterprise." *Yale Law Review* 89 (1980): 835–99.

Harris, J. "The Internal Organization of Hospitals: Some Economic Implications." *Bell Journal of Economics* 8 (1977): 467–82.

Hartz, A., J. Pulido, and E. Kuhn. "Are the Best Coronary Artery Bypass Surgeons Identified by Physician Surveys?" *American Journal of Public Health* 87 (1977): 1645–48.

Hellinger, F. "The Impact of Managed Care on Market Performance: A Review of New Evidence." Mimeo, Agency for Health Care Policy and Research, 1996.

Henry Kaiser Family Foundation/Harvard University/Princeton Survey Research Associates Poll. Storrs, Conn.: Roper Center for Public Opinion Research, 1997.

Hertzlinger, R. *Market-Driven Health Care.* Reading, Mass.: Addison-Wesley, 1997.

Hickson, G., W. Altmeier, and J. Perrin. "Physician Reimbursement by Salary or Fee-for-Service: Effect on Physician Practice Behavior in a Randomized Prospective Study." *Pediatrics* 80 (1987): 344–50.

Hill, S., and B. Wolfe. "Testing the HMO Competitive Strategy." *Journal of Health Economics* 16 (1997): 261–86.

Hillman, B., et al. "Physicians' Utilization and Charges for Outpatient Diagnostic Imaging in a Medicare Population." *Journal of the American Medical Association* 268 (1992): 2050–54.

Hillman, B., et al. "Frequency and Cost of Diagnostic Imaging in Office Practices:

A Comparison of Self-Referring and Radiology-Referring Physicians." *New England Journal of Medicine* 323 (1990): 1604–5.

Hillman, A., M. Pauly, and J. Kerstein. "How Do Financial Incentives Affect Physicians' Clinical Decisions and the Financial Performance of Health Maintenance Organizations?" *New England Journal of Medicine* 321 (1989): 86–92.

Himmelstein, D., et al. "Quality of Care in Investor-Owned vs. Not-for-Profit HMOs." *Journal of the American Medical Association* 282 (1999): 159–63.

Hofer, T., et al. "The Unreliability of Individual Physician 'Report Cards' for Assessing the Costs and Quality of Care for a Chronic Disease." *Journal of the American Medical Association* 281 (1999): 2098–105.

Kao, A., et al. "The Relationship between Method of Physician Payment and Patient Trust." *Journal of the American Medical Association* 280 (1998): 1708–14.

Kaplan, R. "Utility Assessment for Estimating Quality-Adjusted Life Years." In *Valuing Health Care: Costs, Benefits, and Effectiveness of Pharmaceuticals and Other Medical Technologies*, ed. F. Sloan, 31–60. Cambridge: Cambridge University Press, 1995.

Karlan, A. "Rankings Miss Hospitals' Human Side." *Chicago Tribune*, November 10, 1998, sec. 1, p. 26.

Kleinke, J. D. "Release 0.0: Clinical Information Technology in the Real World." *Health Affairs* 17, no. 6 (1992): 23–38.

Laupacis, A., et al. "How Attractive Does a New Technology Have to Be to Warrant Adoption and Utilization?" *Canadian Medical Journal* 146 (1992): 473–81.

Long, M. "A Reconsideration of Economies of Scale in the Health Care Field." *Health Policy* 5 (1985): 25–44.

Lu, M., et al. "Risk Selection and Matching in Performance-Based Contracting." Mimeo, University of Calgary, 1999.

Luft, H. "How Do Health Maintenance Organizations Achieve Their 'Savings'?" *New England Journal of Medicine* 298 (1978): 1336–43.

Luft, H., et al. *Hospital Volume, Physician Volume, and Patient Outcomes: Assessing the Evidence*. Health Administration Press Perspectives. Ann Arbor, Mich.: Health Administration Press, 1990.

Lyman, R. "Public Rights and Private Responsibilities: A University Viewpoint." *Journal of Medical Education* 51 (1976): 9.

Lynk, W. "The Creation of Economic Efficiencies in Hospital Mergers." *Journal of Health Economics* 14 (1995): 507–30.

Management Strategies Used by Large Employers to Control Costs. U.S. General Accounting Office Report 97–71. Washington, D.C.: U.S. General Accounting Office, 1997.

Manning, W., et al. "A Controlled Trial of the Effect of a Prepaid Group Practice on the Use of Services." *New England Journal of Medicine* 310 (1984): 1505–10.

Mayer, T., and G. Mayer. "HMOs: Origins and Development." *New England Journal of Medicine* 312 (1985): 590–94.

Mechanic, D. "Changing Medical Organization and the Erosion of Trust." *Millbank Quarterly* 74 (1996): 171–89.

Mechanic, D. "The Functions and Limitations of Trust in the Provision of Medical Care." *Journal of Health Politics, Policy, and Law* 23 (1998): 661–86.

Melnick, G., et al. "The Effects of Market Structure and Bargaining Position on Hospital Prices." *Journal of Health Economics* 11 (1992): 217–33.

Mennemeyer, S., M. Morrisey, and L. Howard. "Death and Reputation: How Consumers Acted upon HCFA Mortality Information." *Inquiry* 34 (1997): 117–28.

Millenson, M. *Demanding Medical Excellence*. Chicago: University of Chicago Press, 1997.

Miller, I. *American Health Care Blues*. New Brunswick, N.J.: Transaction, 1996.

Miller, R., and H. Luft. "Managed Care Plan Performance since 1980: A Literature Analysis." *Journal of the American Medical Association* 271 (1994): 1512–17.

———. "Managed Care Performance: Is Quality of Care Better or Worse?" *Health Affairs* 16, no. 5 (1997): 7–25.

Miller, W. Letter. *Hospitals*, July 1, 1967.

Mittler, B. "The Demise of the SuperMeds." *Best's Review—Life Insurance Edition* 87 (1987): 50.

Moore, J. "Med School Applicants Drop Again." *Modern Healthcare*, September 12, 1999, 26.

Morrisey, M. *Cost-Shifting in Healthcare: Separating Evidence from Rhetoric*. Washington, D.C.: American Enterprise Institute, 1994.

———. "State Health Care Reform: Protecting the Provider." In *American Health Care: Government, Market Processes, and the Public Interest*, ed. M. Morrisey. Oakland, Calif.: The Independent Institute, 1999.

Morrisey, M., F. Sloan, and J. Valvona. "Medicare Prospective Payment and Posthospital Transfers." *Medical Care* 26 (1998): 685–98.

Morrisey, M. A., G. J. Wedig, and M. Hassan. "Do Non-profit Hospitals Pay Their Way?" *Health Affairs* 15, no. 4 (1996): 132–44.

Moskowitz, D. "Coloradians Tame the Guidelines Beast." *Business and Health* 16, no. 10 (1998): 63–64.

Mukamel, D., and A. Mushlin. "Quality of Care Information Makes a Difference." *Medical Care* 36 (1998): 945–54.

Newhouse, J. "Toward a Theory of Nonprofit Institutions: An Economic Model of a Hospital." *American Economic Review* 60 (1970): 64–74.

Noether, M. "The Effect of Government Policy Changes on the Supply of Physicians: Expansion of a Competitive Fringe." *Journal of Law and Economics* 29 (1986): 231–62.

O'Conner, G., et al. "Geographic Variation in the Treatment of Acute Myocardial Infarction: The Cooperative Cardiovascular Project." *Journal of the American Medical Association* 281 (1999): 627–33.

Office of Inspector General. *Financial Arrangements between Physicians and Health Care Businesses*. Washington, D.C.: Department of Health and Human Services, 1989.

Pantilat, C., M. Chesney, and B. Lo. "Effect of Incentives on the Use of Indicated Services in Managed Care." *Western Journal of Medicine* 170 (1999): 137–42.

Pattison, R., and H. Katz. "Investor-Owned and Not-for-Profit Hospitals: A Comparison Based on California Data." *New England Journal of Medicine* 309 (1982): 347–53.

Pauly, M. *Doctors and Their Workshops.* Chicago: University of Chicago Press, 1980.

Pauly, M., and M. Redisch. "The Not-for-Profit Hospital as a Physicians' Cooperative." *American Economic Review* 63 (1973): 87–99.

Phelps, C. "Induced Demand—Can We Ever Know Its Extent?" *Journal of Health Economics* 5 (1986): 355–65.

———. *Health Economics.* Reading, Mass.: Addison-Wesley, 1997.

Phelps, C., and C. Mooney. "Variations in Medical Practice Use: Causes and Consequences." In *Competitive Approaches to Health Care Reform,* ed. D. Arnould, R. Rich, and W. White. Washington, D.C.: Urban Institute Press, 1993.

Phelps, C., et al. "Doctors Have Styles—and They Matter!" University of Rochester working paper, 1994.

"Prescription for Profits: Private Hospital Firms Bring Management Skills to the Bedside." *Time,* July 4, 1983, 42.

Ramsey, J. "A Re-evaluation of Supply and Demand Concepts in Physician Care." Report submitted to the Department of Health and Human Services, contract No. HRA 79-0068, 1981.

Relman, A. "The New Medical-Industrial Complex." *New England Journal of Medicine* 303 (1980): 963.

Riley, G., et al. "Stage at Diagnosis and Treatment Patterns among Older Women with Breast Cancer: An HMO and Fee-for-Service Comparison." *Journal of the American Medical Association* 281 (1999): 720–26.

Robinson, J. "Vertical Integration and Organizational Networks in Health Care." *Health Affairs* 15, no. 1 (1996): 7–22.

Robinson, J., and H. Luft. "The Impact of Hospital Market Structure on Patient Volume, Average Length of Stay, and the Cost of Care." *Journal of Health Economics* 4 (1985): 333–56.

Roemer, M. "Bed Supply and Hospital Utilization: A Natural Experiment." *Hospitals* 35 (1961): 36–42.

Rosenblatt, R., and A. Rubin. "Lag in Health Tests for Medicare Patients Found." *Buffalo News,* April 19, 1999. 4A.

Salkever, D., and T. Bice. "The Impact of Certificate of Need Controls on Hospital Investment." *Milbank Quarterly* 54 (1976): 185–214.

Sandrick, K. "Out in Front: Managed Care Helps Push Clinical Guidelines Forward." *Hospitals* 67, no. 9 (1993): 30–31.

Schauffler, H., C. Brown, and A. Milstein. "Raising the Bar: The Use of Performance Guarantees by the Pacific Business Group on Health." *Health Affairs* 18 (1999): 11 134–42.

Schneider, E., and A. Epstein. "Influence of Cardiac-Surgery Performance Reports on Referral Practices and Access to Care: A Survey of Cardiovascular Specialists." *New England Journal of Medicine* 335 (1996): 251–56.

Schnelle, J., et al. "Objective and Subjective Measures of the Quality of Managed Care in Nursing Homes." *Medical Care* 37 (1999): 375–83.

Schwartz, A., D. Colby, and A. Reisinger. "Variation in Medicaid Physician Fees." *Health Affairs* 10 (spring 1991): 131–39.

Scitovsky, A., and N. McCall. "Coinsurance and the Demand for Physician Services: Four Years Later." *Social Security Bulletin* 35, no. 6 (1977): 3–19.

Scott-Morton, F. "The Strategic Response by Pharmaceutical Firms to the Medicaid Most-Favored-Customer Rules." *RAND Journal of Economics* 28 (1997): 269–90.

Seidman, J., et al. "Review of Studies that Compare the Quality of Cardiovascular Care in HMO versus Non-HMO Settings." *Medical Care* 36 (1998): 1607–20.

Shortell, S. *A Model of Physician Referral Behavior: A Test of Exchange Theory in Medical Practice*. Chicago: University of Chicago Center for Health Administration Studies Research Series no. 31, 1973.

Shortell, S., et al. "Assessing the Impact of Continuous Quality Improvement on Clinical Practice: What It Will Take to Accelerate Progress." *Milbank Quarterly* 76 (1998): 593–625.

Simon, C., D. Dranove, and W. White. "The Impact of Managed Care on the Physician Marketplace." *Public Health Reports* 112 (1997): 222–30.

Sirower, M. *The Synergy Trap*. New York: Free Press, 1997.

Sisk, J. "How Are Health Care Organizations Using Clinical Guidelines?" *Health Affairs* 17, no. 5 (1998): 91–109.

Sloan, F. "Rate Regulation as a Strategy for Hospital Cost Control." *Milbank Memorial Fund Quarterly* 61 (1983): 195–221.

Sloan, F., and R. Vraciu. "Investor-Owned and Not-for-Profit Hospitals: Addressing Some Issues." *Health Affairs* 2 (spring 1983): 25–34.

Sloan, F., et al. "Hospital Ownership and Cost and Quality of Care: Is There a Dime's Worth of Difference?" National Bureau of Economic Research, working paper 6706, 1998.

Somers, A., and H. Somers, eds. *Health and Health Care: Policies in Perspective*. Germantown, Md.: Aspen, 1977.

Soumerai, T., et al. "Timeliness and Quality of Care for Elderly Patients with Acute Myocardial Infarction under Health Maintenance Organizations vs. Fee-for-Service Insurance." *Archives of Internal Medicine* 159 (1999): 2013–20.

Starr, P. *The Social Transformation of American Medicine*. New York: Basic Books, 1982.

Steering Committee on Clinical Practice Guidelines for the Care and Treatment of Breast Cancer. "Adjuvant Systematic Therapy for Women with Node-Positive Breast Cancer." *Canadian Medical Association Journal* 158, S3 (1998): S52–S64.

Stern, S., and M. Trajtenberg. "Empirical Implications of Physician Authority in Pharmaceutical Decision Making." National Bureau of Economic Research, working paper 6851, 1998.

Stevens, R. *Welfare Medicine in America*. New York: Free Press, 1994.

"Summary Report of the Graduate Medical Education National Advisory Committee to the Secretary, Department of Health and Human Services." DHHS Publication no. (HRA) 81–651. Washington, D.C.: U.S. Department of Health and Human Services, 1980.

Sussman, E., and K. Langa. "The Effect of Cost-Containment Policies on Rates of Coronary Revascularization in California." *New England Journal of Medicine* 329 (1993): 1784–89.

Thaler, R., and S. Rosen. "The Value of Saving a Life: Evidence from the Labor Market." In *Household Production and Consumption*, ed. N. Terlecky. New York: National Bureau of Economic Research, 1975.

Tolley, G., D. Kenkel, and R. Fabian. *Valuing Health for Policy: An Economic Approach*. Chicago: University of Chicago Press, 1994.

Ullman, M., et al. "Performance Measurement in Prostate Cancer Care: Beyond Report Cards." *Urology* 47 (1996): 356–65.

Viscusi, W. K. "The Value of Risks to Life and Health." *Journal of Economic Literature* 31 (1993): 1912–46.

Ware J., and C. Sherbourne. "The MOS 36-Item Short-Form Health Survey (SF-36): I. Conceptual Framework and Item Selection." *Medical Care* 30 (1992): 473–83.

Ware, J., et al. "Differences in 4-Year Health Outcomes for Elderly and Poor, Chronically Ill Patients Treated in HMO and Fee-for-Service Systems." *Journal of the American Medical Association* 276 (1996): 1039–40.

Watt, J., et al. "The Comparative Economic Performance of Investor-Owned Chain and Not-for-Profit Hospitals." *New England Journal of Medicine* 314 (1986): 89–96.

Weinstein, M. "Managed Care's Other Problem: It's Not What You Think." *New York Times*, February 4, 1999, sec. 4, pp. 1, 4.

Weisbrod, B. *The Nonprofit Economy*. Cambridge, Mass.: Harvard University Press, 1988.

———. "The Health Care Quadrilemma: An Essay on Technological Change, Insurance, Quality of Care, and Cost Containment." *Journal of Economic Literature* 29 (1991): 523–52.

Weissman, J., et al. "Market Forces and Unsponsored Research in Academic Health Centers." *Journal of the American Medical Association* 281 (1999): 1093–98.

Wennberg, J., J. Freeman, and W. Culp. "Are Hospital Services Rationed in New Haven or Over-utilised in Boston?" *Lancet* 1 (1987): 1185–88.

White House Domestic Policy Council. *Health Security: The President's Report to the American People*. 1993, 62.

Wickizer, T., and D. Lessler. "Do Treatment Restrictions Imposed by Utilization Management Increase the Likelihood of Readmission for Psychiatric Patients?" *Medical Care* 36 (1998): 844–50.

Wickizer, T., J. Wheeler, and P. Feldstein. "Does Utilization Review Reduce Unnecessary Hospital Care and Contain Costs?" *Medical Care* 27 (1989): 632–47.

Williams, G. *Kaiser-Permanente Health Plan: Why It Works*. Oakland, Calif.: Kaiser Foundation, 1991.

Williams, S., and P. Torrens. *Introduction to Health Services*. New York: Wiley, 1988.

Winslow, R. "Heart Attack Therapy Varies Sharply by Region." *Wall Street Journal*, February 17, 1999, B5.

———. "Elderly Need Preventive Care but Don't Get It." *Wall Street Journal*, April 19, 1999, sec. 2, p. B4.

Wynia, M., D. Cummins, and J. VanGeest. "Physician Responses to Utilization

Review Pressures: Results of a National Survey." Chicago: AMA Institute for Ethics, 1999.

Yip, W. "Physician Response to Medicare Fee Reductions: Changes in the Volume of Coronary Artery Bypass Graft Surgeries in the Medicare and Private Sectors." *Journal of Health Economics* 17 (1998): 675–700.

Zwanziger, J., and A. Meirowitz. "Strategic Factors in Hospital Selection for HMO and PPO Networks." In *Managed Care and Chaning Health Care Markets*, ed. M. Morrisey. Washington, D.C.: American Enterprise Institute, 1998.

Index

accreditation, of hospitals, 144–45, 154
activity-based cost accounting (ABC), 112, 167
AdMar, 70, 71
Advocate hospital system (Chicago), 115
Aetna Insurance, 20, 127, 128, 153
age, of physicians, 104–5
Agency for Healthcare Research and Quality (AHRQ), 99
agents: government as, 61–62; health maintenance organizations as, 41; and uncertainty in decision-making, 14
allocation, of health resources, 141–43
American Hospital Asociation, 115
American Medical Association (AMA), 16, 38, 39, 67, 98–99, 126
American Medical International (AMI), 58, 59
America's Health Network, 149
Anthem Blue Cross and Blue Shield, 152–53
antitrust cases: and hospital mergers, 123–25, 126; and managed care mergers, 172; and physicians' groups, 161
any willing provider (AWP) legislation, 71
Archives of Internal Medicine, 99
Arrow, Kenneth, 9–10, 11–12, 20, 31, 39, 93, 143
Association of American Medical Colleges, 54
assurance, and nonprofit health care providers, 23–24
autonomy, of physicians, 19–20

Balachandran, Bala, 112
Bayesian statistics, 168
Berman, Joseph, 146
beta-blockers, 79, 138
Bice, T., 182n.23
BJC hospital system (St. Louis), 116, 187n.1
Blue Choice HMO (St. Louis), 153
Blue Cross and Blue Shield: beginning of, 37–38; and cost-based reimbursement, 46; medical records and measurement of costs, 113; as nonprofits, 21; and pre-

ferred provider organizations, 71; and promotion of health maintenance organizations, 66–67; and purchasing power, 127
bounded rationality, 15
branding strategies: and for-profit health care, 60–61; and pharmacy benefits management, 108. *See also* differentiation
breast cancer, 98. *See also* mammograms
British National Health Service. *See* Great Britain
Brook, Robert, 17, 137, 138
Brown, Catherine, 157
Brown, Fred, 119
Buchmueller, Thomas, 187n.23
Bunker, John, 137
Business Health Care Action Group (BHCAG), 68
business management, and physicians, 104–5

California: and legislation on PPOs, 70–71; and Medicaid cutbacks, 51
Campbell, Thomas, 161
Canada: and per capita spending on health care, 28, 63; and quality adjusted life years, 142; and regional referral centers, 103
capital markets, and nonprofit health care providers, 22–23
capitation, and primary care physicians, 75–76
Cassel, Christine, 80
causality, and demand inducement, 34–35, 179n.9
Center for Healthcare Industry Performance Studies (CHIPS), 149
centers of excellence, 102–3
Cerezyme, 108
certificate-of-need (CON) laws, 55–56
charity, and nonprofit health care providers, 21
Chernew, Michael, 86
Chicago Tribune, 143, 168
Cleary, P. D., 191n.4
Cleveland Clinic, 168–69